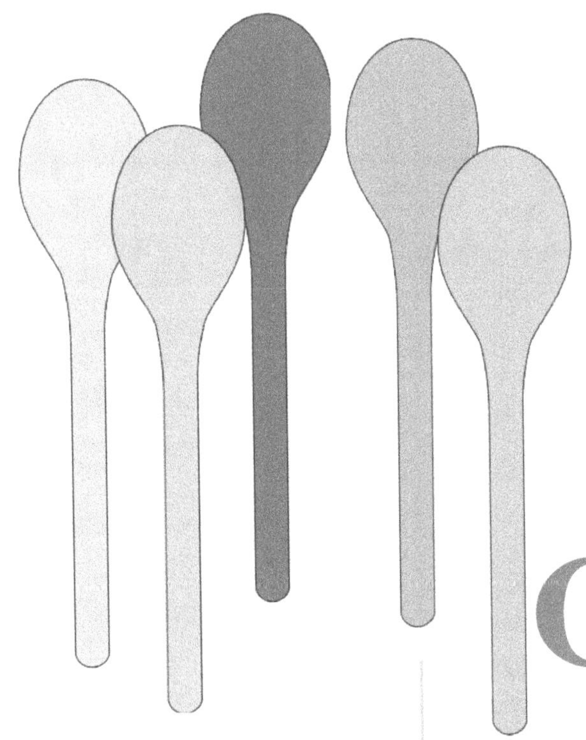

Fun with Gluten-Free, Low Glycemic Food Cookbook

Rich, delicious food you can eat!

Acknowledgments

Without these people, I would not know what I do about cooking and eating fabulously healthy, yet delicious food.

In memory of my mom, who was such an incredible baker that the neighbor ladies begged her to teach a class. Bless her for dragging me down from whatever tree I was climbing to make me watch and help her bake delicious desserts.

Thank you, college roommates, for teaching me to make things I'd never heard of and to eat Jello with chopsticks. (Yes, that's relevant, it contributed to my belief that I could do anything with food!!)

Thank you, old boyfriends, for teaching me various ethnic cooking, from crêpes to salsa.

Thank you, good friends, who have fed me and expanded my vision of what was possible with food.

Thank you, Shyrl, for your editing help.

Thank you, Sunni, for more editing (can you believe I really kept goofing things up!), as well as your incredible, beautiful design work. I love the new look!

Thank you, John Houlgate, for your patient, kind and continuous help with both this book and my Web site.

Thank you, God and Divine Spirit, for giving me whatever creative abilities I have and for guiding me in this work, to work in six parts of my brain at the same time to create food that can be eaten by just about anyone. Yay team!

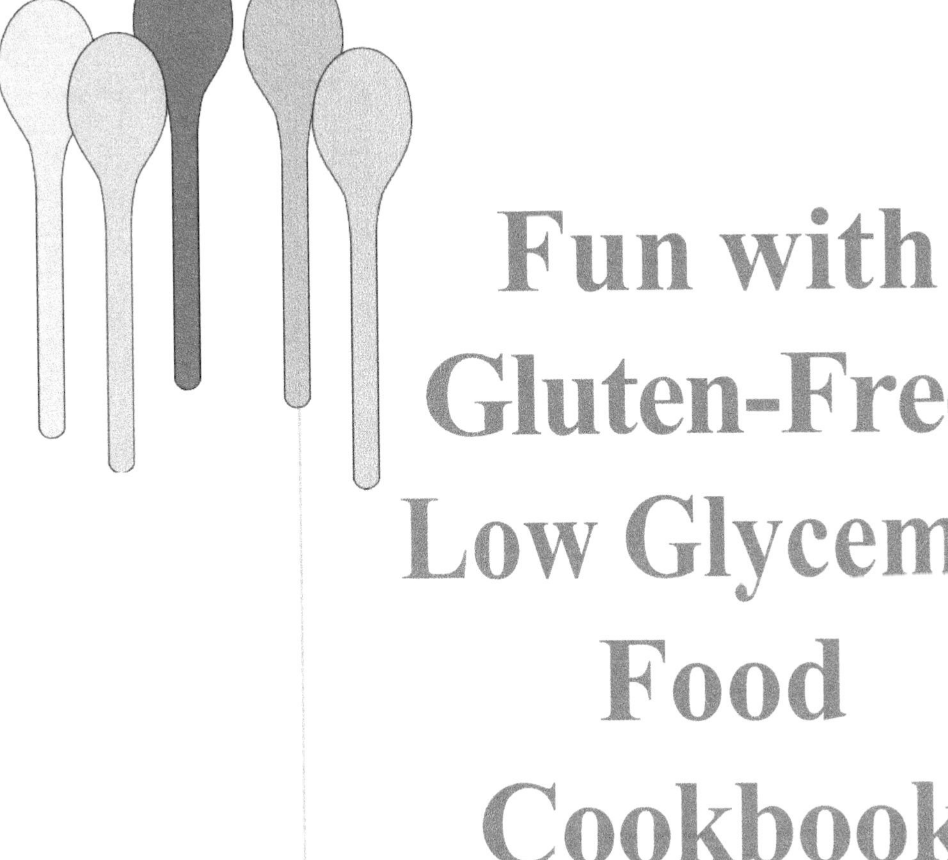

Fun with Gluten-Free, Low Glycemic Food Cookbook

Rich, delicious food you can eat!

Debbie Johnson

Fun with Gluten-Free, Low Glycemic Food Cookbook
©Copyright June 2008
Deborah A. Johnson
Deborah Johnson Publishing

Deborah Johnson Publishing, glutenfreefun@gmail.com.

To get a copy of this book go to:

https://debbiejohnsonbooks.com/gluten-free-low-carb-cookbooks.

Important Disclaimer

Consult your doctor for which recipes or variations of recipes are acceptable for your health condition. Also, we cannot be held responsible for your source of ingredients. Please read all labels and check with your doctor about any ingredients used.

Contents

Restaurants or other Food Establishments wishing to use any of these recipes must purchase them for $500.00 each. Call 800-600-3483 for a licensing agreement.

Important Disclaimer

Everyone's body chemistry is unique and therefore you must check with your doctor before using any of these recipes. We will not be held legally responsible for any response your body has to them. Please check all labels on food and sources. We cannot be held responsible for your source of ingredients.

Introduction

People Loved the Food at My Restaurant

After experimenting for about 20 years with making healthy food taste rich, satisfying and flavorful, I opened my restaurant. I wanted to cook for those who needed to eat gluten-free as well as low-glycemic. I called it **The Golden Chalice** because I wanted it to be the holy grail of delicious, heavenly, healthy food for all, no matter what the allergy or health challenge might be. I made the environment completely safe, from no-VOC paint and recycled carpeting to chemical-free cleaners.

Recipe titles beginning with the words **"Golden Chalice"** were on the menu at my restaurant and well-loved by our guests.

I truly believe that eating the way I have, mostly gluten-free and very low-glycemic, has kept me younger, stronger and healthier than I would have been otherwise. The interesting thing is I really don't want to eat any other way. It doesn't even look good to me anymore! It actually disgusts me to think of eating a sugar-coated donut. You know what I mean if you've been eating really clean for a few years.

After spending decades to make health foods yummy, and it was a blast for me to do so, I hope you enjoy the recipes in this book.

Very Special Ingredients in Our Restaurant Foods and in this Book

Just as the health of my restaurant guests was very important to me, so is the health of my readers. It's a matter of integrity. I love to help people make their dreams come true, whether in health, business or personal success. And of course, good health is required for it all of the above.

The ingredients in every single recipe have been carefully chosen for your optimal health. They are not only good for you in the nutritional sense, according to experts, they are also healing foods. You will find these foods in nearly every book on healing, including books (*Alkalize or Die*, *pH Miracle*, etc.) on alkalizing your body for optimum health.

I have also taken great care to exclude possible allergens (no gluten, no refined sugar, no corn, no soy).

Exceptions: There are some milk, tree nut and soy products for which I have given alternatives. Also, I recommend Braggs Liquid Amino Acids (like soy sauce) quite a bit since it is a well-broken down gluten-free, non-GMO soy product that works well for many people.

Each person must check with their doctor for questions on their own sensitivities.

See Appendix A for ingredients specifically left out of recipes and why and see Appendix B for ingredients I do use and why.

You may notice with these recipes that you don't need to eat as much, because you're getting more concentrated nutrition.

Please notice the variations following each recipe. These are new recipes in themselves, as they often create a much different flavor—so you're getting many more recipes as my gift to you. The more you eat these food combinations, the more you may find yourself wanting them. I know I have.

I sincerely hope you will enjoy these recipes and will be creative enough to develop your own based on them.

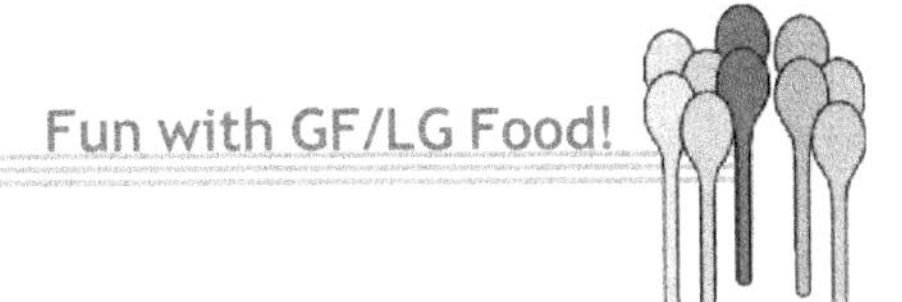

Chapter 1
Simple Prep
and Starters

Simplifying the Prep Process

Delegate! If you're cooking for a family, and you have children old enough to tear lettuce, you can engage their help. I was helping make salads from the age of eight and was cooking dinner for my family at thirteen. I had to. My mother worked. Kids can do so much more than we think they can. I have a degree in elementary education and I did Montessori training post-grad. I've seen kids do amazing things when they were trusted.

If you don't have children old enough or another housemate or family member willing to help, you can buy many pre-packaged, pre-washed organic fruits and vegetables, as well as ground Almonds, a staple in much of the baking in this book. These are the more labor-intensive things.

If you have a food processor, you can certainly do some advance veggie chopping and store in green bags found in health food stores to keep things fresher longer.

Success Secrets

Here are a few **Success Secrets** to get you started. You'll find lots more of these sprinkled generously throughout this book.

Success Secret: Organic ingredients are always recommended. The flavor is superior and you need less in the way of "dressing up" such as sauces or spices. Many gourmet restaurants now use organic ingredients as a matter of taste and pride.

Organic is likely better for your health as well as the health of the planet. Again, check with a doctor you trust. Eating organic is the only way you can be assured of non-GMO (genetically modified) foods as well as little or no use of harmful chemicals that may be damaging to the health of someone whose body is already stressed with allergies and sensitivities.

I know that eating organic is a little more expensive, but think of what your life or the life of your loved one is worth. You can spend more now or more later, but if you wait until it's too late, the quality of life has already been compromised. And you're donating to a good cause, helping the environment by eating organically contributes to its cleanliness and sustainability.

Every recipe in this book has some kind of "healing" food, according to many books written by doctors who are experts in the field of nutrition.

The rule of thumb to help you make every single thing you eat taste great is to use totally natural ingredients, made from scratch, with healthy, raw or cold-pressed oils and fresh, organic herbs and spices.

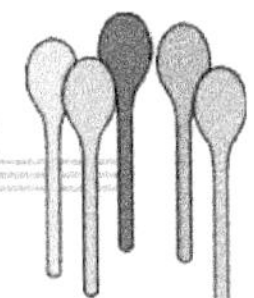

Success Secret: I keep my herbs and spices in the freezer until use and they have all the flavor they did when fresh! Fresh flavor offers gourmet taste.

Health food stores with produce sections will have all you need to get started. If they don't have what you need, many stores will be happy to special order things that are in bottles or cans. Some produce may not be available in smaller towns, but you can substitute more of the other items in the recipe.

Success Secret: Taste everything before you finish. Make sure it tastes the way you want it to! Herbs and spices may lose some flavor after sitting in your cupboard for a while— that's why I freeze them.

Success Secret: Freshly ground spices and herbs taste so much better. They really make the meal. Try grating dried, whole organic nutmeg or grinding organic cinnamon sticks, broken into pieces, in your coffee grinder.

Success Secret: If you want to cook with oil, the healthiest and most flavorful way is naturally derived oils that have a high heat tolerance. They are called "high flash-point" or "high heat" oils because they don't turn rancid as easily upon heating. Avoid olive oil for cooking as it has the lowest flash point. Use it instead as an after-garnish or in salad dressings. The best cooking oils and fats are, believe it or not, butter (or ghee—clarified butter), bacon grease, grape-seed oil, cold-pressed coconut oil and a new one, high heat sunflower oil.

Soy-sensitive people: NON-SOY users who want an alternative to Bragg Aminos (my soy sauce alternative, still made with soy) can try Coconut Aminos. Ingredients are: organic coconut sap aged and blended with sun dried, mineral rich sea salt; 1 tsp has 1 gram of carbohydrates. Coconut Aminos taste like soy sauce to most people. Find it at health food stores or Coconut Secret at *http://www.coconutsecret.com* and 888-369-3393.

Important Note for Special Dietary Needs and Changing Favorite Recipes from Other Books/Sources

To adapt any of your favorite recipes, experiment with the recipes in this book first, then simply test the ideas with your favorite foods. Here are some examples:

Use vegetables to replace starchy foods like crackers or chips—use Veggie Chips (p. 8) in place of grain chips for dips and spreads.

In place of pasta, try julienne vegetables (p. 69), like in Stroganoff. Use julienne zucchini and other neutral tasting veggies in place of noodles. Some bits of cooked egg may give it a richer flavor, as if using egg noodles.

Instead of flour, use ground nuts and/or seeds plus ¼ cup seed-type flour such as amaranth or quinoa (see dessert section) which will work with nearly any recipe except cookies, unless you use about ½ tsp starch or more for larger recipes, to hold them together. You can get arrowroot powder at your local health food store, or they may order it for you.

For sweetener that tastes like sugar and is unrefined, use Unsweetened Apple Sauce plus sweet leaf stevia. Double the Unsweetened Apple Sauce for the sugar in recipe, then add ½ tsp sweet leaf stevia (or other form of stevia, to taste) per cup of Unsweetened Apple Sauce to sweeten anything from cakes to pies—and lower the liquid level. The tough challenge is in finding a good sprouted bread, but we've got one in the snack chapter, Sprouted Soufflé Flatbread (p. 102).

Special Note for Desperation Dinners and Bare Cupboards

Use what you've got! If you don't have all the ingredients, use whatever seems good. That should be a neutral flavor or one that seems to fit the bill. And be sure to add lots of flavor by using the herbs recommended or similar ones. Be creative as you wish...I came up with these recipes because I didn't always have what I needed and it usually became a new recipe!

Please Note: Results of these recipes will vary according to ingredients used, as many fresh ingredients will have variations of flavor, texture, etc. Please experiment in your own way to find what works best for you. I do consult for people on cooking for special diets and will certainly help you with anything you question in this book. Just contact me at *http://glutenfreefun.com*

Most Important of All: Have Fun and Cook with Love, the Best Ingredient of All!

Starters

Let's get started with the healthiest, yet most ignored of all foods, Vegetables! Here you will find them resplendent in all their glory, from root vegetables to legumes, made to delight the senses—from the visual to the palate.

If you want to be fed with health-giving, easily digestible foods, you've come to the right place!

Recipes beginning with the words *"Golden Chalice"* are from my former gluten-free, diabetic-friendly restaurant of the same name.

Variations

- Instead of Oregano, use organic Tarragon.
- Instead of Oregano, use organic Rosemary.
- Instead of Oregano, use organic Basil.

Note: For this recipe, dried Herbs are best unless you use very finely cut fresh Herbs and soak in Lemon Water for 24 hours before adding Veggies.

Golden Chalice
CRUDITÉS

As an introduction to a meal, while your guests are waiting to be served the initial soup, salad or other appetizer, you can offer them a delightful, simple treat some countries serve as a tradition.

Serves: Varies

Ingredients:
    Assorted vegetables
    Carrots
    Celery
    String Beans
    Bok Choy
    Red Bell Pepper
    Orange and/or Yellow Bell Peppers
    Purified Water to cover Veggies
    Juice of ½ organic Lemon per cup of Water
    1 tsp organic Oregano per cup of Water

1. Choose fresh, crisp organic Vegetables that will slice easily into sticks.
2. Slice into sticks and marinate for four hours or more (24 hours at most) in a mixture of the Water, Lemon Juice and Oregano.

Success Secret: When you have a creative inspiration, test a small amount first so that you don't have to start all over if it doesn't taste as good as you thought it would. For example, take out one tablespoon or soup, spread or main dish, then add a small bit of the herb or ingredient you think might work and taste it!

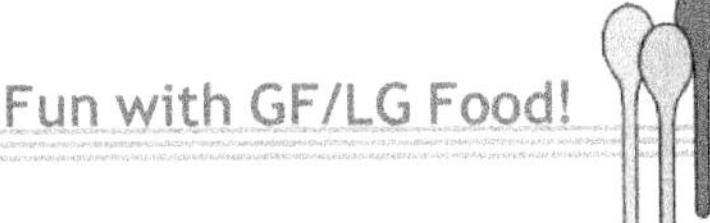

Variations

- Instead of Roasted Red Pepper, add ¼ cup chopped Kalamata Olives, organic or natural with no chemical additives. Add more if you like a stronger olive taste.
- Instead of Roasted Red Pepper, add ¼ cup organic toasted Sesame Seeds or other freshly toasted seeds or nuts. Very satisfying!
- Instead of Roasted Red Pepper, add organic Artichoke Hearts, preferably bottled (not canned) and not marinated.

Success Secret: Mix crunchy with smooth, salty with sweet. Opposite balances make for tastier treats.

Golden Chalice ROASTED-RED-PEPPER HUMMUS

This flavorful garbanzo bean dip or spread is so filling it can be served as a meal in itself with other starters such as soup and salad.

Serves: Six people for an appetizer or three for a small meal

Ingredients:

1 cup organic Garbanzo Beans
    or to simplify, 2 cups canned organic Garbanzo beans
    (no need to cook further if canned)
¼ tsp Celtic Sea Salt
    or ¼ tsp Pink Himalayan Salt
¼ cup purified Water or more for desired consistency
1 organic Red Bell Pepper, seeded and cut into squares
2 Tbsp. organic Tahini
    (Sesame Seed Butter—health food section/store)
¼ cup chopped organic Parsley
2 Tbsp. organic Lemon Juice
2 Tbsp. organic Olive Oil
1 clove crushed organic Garlic

1. Soak Garbanzo Beans overnight in 3 cups purified Water, unless using canned.
2. Rinse and cook the soaked Beans in 3 cups purified Water with the Salt for 4 hours or until very soft.
3. While Beans are cooking, you can prepare the rest of the recipe. Roast Peppers at 350 °F in oven for about 10 minutes or until soft. You can also roast on grill.
4. Blend all ingredients in blender until smooth, reserving small amount of roasted Pepper for garnish, if you wish.
5. Spread your hummus on raw, gluten-free sprouted Flaxseed and Veggie Crackers or gluten-free Almond Crackers, or better yet, use the Veggie Chip recipe idea (p. 8) for dipping instead of chips as the low-glycemic choice. If I really want Chips or Crackers, I sometimes use a combination of both the Veggie Chips and gluten-free Crackers. That way I'm not getting as many complex carbs.

Golden Chalice
VEGGIE "CHIPS"

If you really want to have greater health and follow the dictums of every doctor, health practitioner, article, study and even the AMA, then having more veggies in your is essential. These veggie chips are an excellent way and I find them just as satisfying as chips after the first few bites. They tend to grow on you! (No pun intended.)

Makes: Varies

Ingredients:
Find Veggies in your fridge that are firm enough to slice at an angle to make them bigger and shaped well for dipping. Carrots are my favorite for Guacamole (p. 9) because the sweet flavor seems almost like corn chips to me.

Suggestions:

Carrots	Bok Choy	Chinese Cabbage
Sugar Snap Pea-Pods	Zucchini	Cucumber
Celery	Red Cabbage	Turnip
Radish		

1. I'd recommend slicing the Vegetables about ¼-inch thick or thick enough to be sure they are firm for dipping or spreading upon.
2. For the Cabbage, simply cut in triangles to dip or squares big enough to use like a cracker upon which to spread.
3. The Snap Peas can be cut in half to better catch the dip.

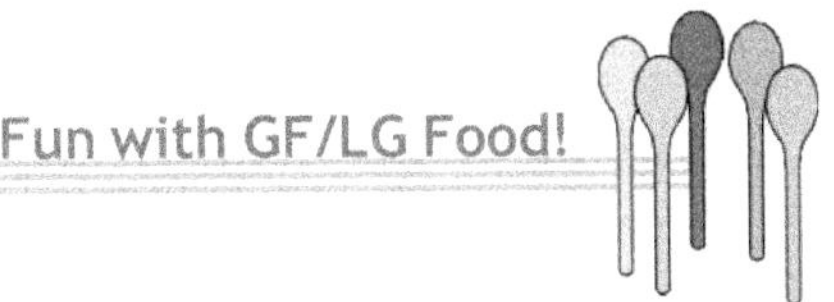

Variations

- For a unique flavor, (and especially for alternative to nightshades), try just adding ¼ tsp Cumin (or more for flavor) instead of Chili Powder or Salsa.
- If you are eating nightshades, add ¼ cup or one small, ripe organic Tomato, cut in ½ inch cubes or smaller.

Vegans and dairy- or soy-sensitive people:

Replace the Sour Cream with Savory Cashew Cream or for tree-nut allergies, use ground Flaxseed or Chia Seeds mixed half and half in water to thicken anything.

Golden Chalice GUACAMOLE

This classic Mexican dish can also become a meal with some hearty flaxseed crackers or even as a sandwich spread if you can eat sprouted seed and grain bread. Most of that sort of bread contains Wheat as the first ingredient, but since it's sprouted, it has much less gluten. If you have Celiac disease you should avoid it. It is, however, very low glycemic for those who are most concerned about that piece and can also eat soy, as most sprouted grain breads have soy as well.

Serves: Two people

Ingredients:
- 1 organic Avocado
- 1 Tbsp. freshly grated or finely chopped organic Onion 1 Tbsp. fresh squeezed organic Lemon Juice
    (even bottled organic doesn't taste as good)
- $1/_8$ tsp organic Cumin
- ½ tsp organic Chili Powder,
    or 1 Tbsp. of your favorite organic Salsa
- ¼ tsp Celtic Sea Salt
    ¼ tsp or Pink Himalayan Salt
- 1 Tbsp. Sour Cream (optional)
    or 1 Tbsp. Goat Cheese
    or 1 Tbsp. Savory Cashew Cream (p. 14, 15 or 40)
    or for tree-nut allergies, use ground Flaxseed or Chia

1. Mash Avocado with a fork. Add and mash in rest of ingredients.
2. If you want a smoother flavor, add organic cultured Sour Cream or if you prefer, soft Goat Cheese (better for you and easier on the system).
3. Serve in bowl with lots of veggie chips described above. Carrots are best because their sweetness mimics what we are used to in corn chips with Avocado dips.

Soy-sensitive people:
Replace Braggs Liquid Amino Acids with Celtic Sea Salt or Pink Himalayan Salt.

Golden Chalice
CURRIED SUNFLOWER PATÉ

This recipe is loaded with nutrients, but much more so if you are sure to soak the sunflower seeds as directed.

Serves: Two to three people

Ingredients:

¼ cup organic Sunflower Seeds, germinated
   (soaked in purified Water for 4-8 hours, rinsed well daily and used within two days—will be about ⅓ cup after soaking)
¼ tsp organic Curry Powder
¼ tsp organic Cumin
½ tsp Braggs Liquid Amino Acids
   or $^1/_{16}$ tsp Celtic Sea Salt
   or $^1/_{16}$ tsp Pink Himalayan Salt

1. Blend all the above in blender or food processor.
2. Serve in bowl or shaped on a plate in whatever fashion you like, along with sprouted flaxseed and vegetable Crackers (health food store—raw section) or veggie Chips (p. 8), but cut some Veggies in cracker-size squares, such as the Chinese Cabbage, especially the thick part of the leaf, and the Red Cabbage. If you have large Carrots, cut them at an angle, such as you see in Chinese food, and they may be good for spreading on as well. Also, Celery, about four inches in length, can hold the dip nicely. Raw Yams, sliced thinly, make a nice bed for this flavor as well.

Success Secret: To stay on a gluten-free, low-glycemic diet requires filling, satisfying food that gives your body all it needs. I find that when I eat Nuts and Seeds, soaked and germinated or roasted, my body feels very satisfied. It may fulfill the Oils and fats I'm not getting with all that Butter I loved on my bread! Our nervous systems need the naturally derived Oils very much, some people more than others.

Variations

- Add 2 Tbsp. of your favorite organic Mexican Salsa instead of Cumin and/or Chili Powder unless you like it very spicy, then just add Cayenne Red Pepper, to taste.
- Add ¼ cup chopped organic Black Olives.
- Add 1 clove Garlic, crushed.

Dairy-sensitive people: Replace the Sour Cream with Savory Cashew Cream **or, for tree-nut allergies,** thicken anything with ground flax or chia seeds.

BLACK BEAN DIP

If you like bean dip, but want the easiest to digest with the most nutrients, black beans are a great and flavorful alternative.

Serves: Six people for an appetizer or three for a small meal

Ingredients:

    1 cup organic Black Beans
        or 2 cups canned, cooked organic Black Beans
        (if canned, skip steps 1 and 2)
    6 cups purified Water unless using canned beans
    1 Tbsp. Celtic Sea Salt, for cooking Beans
        or 1 Tbsp. Pink Himalayan Salt, for cooking Beans
    2 Tbsp. Braggs Liquid Amino Acids
        or 1 tsp Celtic Sea Salt
        or 1 tsp Pink Himalayan Salt
    ¼ cup organic Onion, chopped finely
    1 tsp organic Cumin, to taste
        or 1 tsp Chili Powder, to taste
    Sour cream, to taste
        or Savory Cashew Cream (p. 14, 15 or 40)

1. Soak beans overnight in 3 cups purified Water. Drain water from Beans after soaking.
2. Rinse Black Beans and cook in 3 cups purified Water with 1 Tbsp. Salt until very soft. Drain all but about ¼ cup Water from Beans after cooking.
3. Blend cooked Beans with Onion and Braggs Liquid Amino Acids or Salt and Spices with about ¼ cup purified Water or as needed to make blender work.
4. If needed, add Water until consistency is what you like for dipping or spreading. If you want a mellower flavor, add Sour Cream.

Success Secret: Taste everything you are cooking during the process. You will learn what to add as you build layers of flavor.

Variations

- Roast Cashews at same temperature, but check them at 10 minutes and stir. May only take 15 minutes.
- Roast Seeds like Pumpkin and/or Sunflower at 350 °F. Check and stir every five minutes. May be done at 10 minutes or less.
- Roast Sesame Seeds for topping on salads or stir-fries at 350 °F, checking and stirring every two minutes. May be done in 5 to 10 minutes.

Golden Chalice TAMARI-FLAVOR ROASTED NUTS OR SEEDS

These sell for big bucks at health food stores, now you can make your own!

Serves: Six people for an appetizer or a meal addition

Ingredients:
- 1 cup Almonds
- 1 Tbsp. or more Braggs Liquid Amino Acids
  - or 1 Tbsp. Tamari
  - or 1 Tbsp. Celtic Salt, to taste
  - or 1 Tbsp. Pink Himalayan Salt, to taste

1. Spread Nuts in glass or porcelain baking dish (not metal).

   Important Note: I burned several batches before finding the secret of using porcelain or glass. This avoids having to remove nuts before pouring on the Braggs.
2. Turn oven to 350 °F and place in oven immediately (no preheating).
3. Bake for 20 minutes. Check at 15 minutes in case they are smaller than normal.

   Important Note: See the variations regarding times for other Nuts and especially Seeds.
4. Pull out of oven and immediately pour on Braggs and stir until Nuts are completely coated. Add more if desired for more salty flavor. Nuts will dry quickly even if you add too much. If using Salt instead of Braggs, pour on now to your taste.
5. After about 10 minutes, they may be served as a warm appetizer, though they have more flavor when cooled completely.

Success Secret: Keep Nuts and Seeds refrigerated or frozen for health (roasted nuts and even raw can become rancid easily) and flavor, especially after roasting.

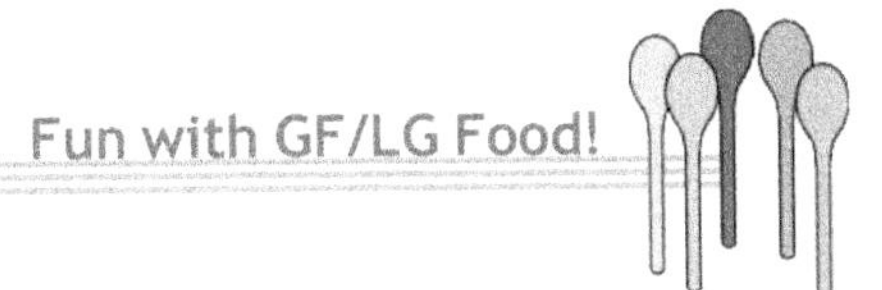

SPROUTED (GERMINATED) NUTS OR SEEDS

Optimal health comes from concentrated, natural nutrition. Any health practitioner will tell you that. One of the easiest ways to get that sort of nutrition is through live, sprouted food. Sprouted almonds are one of the easiest protein sources to digest and absorb, as well as sunflower seeds when sprouted. Pumpkin seeds help kill parasites in the gut, according to some health practitioners.

Serves: Two people for two days as a snack or an addition to meals

Ingredients:
- ½ cup organic Almonds
- ¼ cup organic Sunflower Seeds
- $1/8$ cup organic Pumpkin Seeds
- 3 cups purified Water

1. Place Almonds in quart jar and add 2 cups Water.
2. Place Sunflower and Pumpkin Seeds in separate jar and add 1 cup Water.
3. Leave Sunflower and Pumpkin Seeds to soak for at least 4 hours. Overnight or all day is okay.
4. Leave Almonds overnight or all day and rinse at the end of the day or night. Repeat for another day or night, so they've soaked about 16 hours, or until you see a small "tail" on them.
5. Rinse Nuts and Seeds at end of soak and use immediately, if possible, or within two days, rinsing daily and before each use.

   Important Note: Use sprouted Nuts and Seeds as soon as possible, within two days maximum. They have a tendency to mold otherwise.

SAVORY CASHEW CREAM (Vegan)

When you need cream without sweetness, dairy or soy, here's a raw food alternative. For a yummy dessert, add sweetener and use as garnish for berries or other fruit. See recipe for Sweet Cashew Cream (p. 41 or 80).

Makes: About ¾ cup

Ingredients:
   ½ cup organic Cashews, germinated
       (soaked for eight hours and rinsed well, becomes $^2/_3$ cup
       after soaking—use within two days, rinse daily)
   ¼ cup or more purified Water, depending on preference
   2 dashes Celtic Sea Salt
       or 2 dashes Pink Himalayan Salt

1. Soak Cashews for four more hours in purified Water and rinse well.
2. Blend all ingredients in blender or food processor until smooth.
3. Refrigerate or use immediately. Freeze unused portion within 2 days.

Success Secret: Top chefs agree that fewer ingredients create better flavor. So simple is actually gourmet!

Chapter 2
Super Soups

Why "Super" Soups? Veggies rule in these soups, so they have much more nutritional value than the typical starch-based soup loaded with potatoes or pasta.

Recipes beginning with the words *"Golden Chalice"* are from my former gluten-free, diabetic-friendly restaurant of the same name.

SAVORY CASHEW CREAM (Vegan)

Use in place of sour cream for raw food and dairy-free diets (add lemon juice for sour flavor). You can also use it for other sauces as well as desserts. See Sweet Cashew Cream (p. 41 or 80).

Makes: About ¾ cup

Ingredients:

 ½ cup organic Cashews, germinated
  (soaked for 8 hours and rinsed—becomes ⅔ cup after
  soaking—refrigerate and use within two days, rinse daily)
 ¼ cup purified Water
 2 dashes Celtic Sea Salt
  or 2 dashes Pink Himalayan Salt

1. Blend in blender or food processor until smooth.
2. Refrigerate or use immediately. Freeze unused portion within 2 days.

Variations

- Add other chopped organic Veggies, such as Tomatoes, Celery, Mushrooms or Bok Choy.
- Add to chopped veggies (above) or use alone: raw, organic, soaked (germinated) Nuts and Seeds (p. 13), blended into carrot mixture for added nutrition/protein.
- Add chopped wild-caught Seafood or chopped organic salty Meats that would taste good with a sweet background of Carrots, such as organic Bacon or Turkey Sausage.
- Sprinkle on Dill just before serving (if no other Herbs used).

Dairy- and nut-sensitive people: Add ¼ cup cooked Quinoa to blender for a creamier, milk-like look and taste.

Golden Chalice CREAM OF CARROT SOUP

So simple to make, this soup is inexpensive, yet elegant and delicious with the right seasoning.

Serves: Four to five people

Ingredients:

6 large organic Carrots
4 cups purified Water
2 Tbsp. Braggs Liquid Amino Acids
　or 1 Tbsp. Celtic Sea Salt
　or 1 Tbsp. Pink Himalayan Salt
2 Tbsp. organic Ghee or virgin Coconut Oil
½ large organic Onion
1 cup organic Almond Milk
　or 1 cup organic Goat or Cow's Milk
　or ½ cup organic Cream
　or Savory Cashew Cream (p. 14, 15 or 40)
　or ½ cup organic Quinoa
Seasonings to taste: organic Cumin, Thyme or Rosemary

1. Wash or peel, cut in large chunks and cook Carrots in Water with Braggs Liquid Amino Acids or Salt until soft enough to blend (if you have a Vitamix or strong blending machine, you can do this raw). Add seasonings.
2. While Carrots are cooking, melt Ghee or Coconut Oil. Chop Onion and sauté in Ghee or Oil.
3. Blend Carrots with cooking stock and add sautéed Onions plus Milk or Cream.

Success Secret: When you love the flavor of something, like I do portabella mushrooms, slice thicker than other ingredients for more flavor.

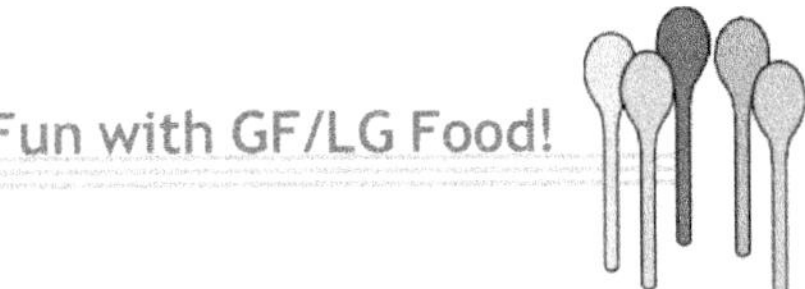

Variations

- Use roasted organic Tomatoes instead of plain.
- Add Dill on top just before serving
- Add Rosemary at the beginning, cooking it in with the Tomatoes and Juice.

Vegans and dairy-sensitive people: Replace the milk with unsweetened Almond Milk or ½ cup organic Cream or Savory Cashew Cream (p. 14, 15 or 40).

Dairy- and nut-sensitive people: Add ¼ cup cooked Quinoa to blender for a creamier, milk-like look and taste.

CREAM OF TOMATO AND MUSHROOM SOUP

This heart-warming, satisfying soup is a real comfort food. I have to credit the invention to my high school boyfriend who heated together a can of Campbell's tomato soup and a can of mushroom soup (before we knew about health food!) and threw it in a thermos when we went skiing. Thank you, Doug!

Serves: Two to four people

Ingredients:

1 16 oz container organic crushed Tomatoes in Juice
1 cup purified Water
2 cups organic sliced Mushrooms
   (Shitake are better for you)
¼ cup Ghee
   or ¼ cup Organic Grape-seed Oil
   or ¼ cup organic high heat Sunflower Oil
¼ cup finely chopped Organic Onion
2 Tbsp. Braggs Liquid Amino Acids, or more to taste
1 cup organic Milk or Milk Substitute of your choice

1. Begin heating Tomatoes and all Liquid in which they were packed with Water and Liquid Amino Acids.
2. Sauté Onions and Mushrooms in Ghee or Oil until cooked and add to Tomato mixture. Heat thoroughly, simmering just slightly so Mushrooms keep their flavor.
3. Add Milk and serve!

Success Secret: Make any soup creamy or thicker by blending either all or part of the finished product when done cooking up to anytime before serving. Or, add cooked grains like Quinoa before blending for heartier texture and to make it more filling. Allow to cool before blending or it may explode in the blender!

Variations

- Add crushed Garlic, one clove.
- Add organic Bacon, crumbled, or Veggie Smoky-flavored Bits.
- Top with organic Sour Cream, Goat Yogurt or Savory Cashew Cream (p. 14, 15 or 40).
- If you can eat night-shades, try organic roasted Red Peppers (p. 7) or organic roasted Tomatoes (available canned).
- Add ¼ cup uncooked, soaked (4-8 hours) organic Quinoa (a higher protein grain)
- Add meat or seafood for higher protein.
- If you want it to taste like chili, just add some organic Chili Powder!

BLACK BEAN AND SQUASH SOUP

This recipe is incredibly versatile and can be easily adapted to your personal tastes. Also, it can be made as only black bean soup, if you prefer. Just leave out the squash. The soup is very versatile and can be like chili as a main meal, too.

Serves: Two to four people

Ingredients:

    1 cup Organic Black Beans (Turtle Beans)
    1 tsp plus 1 pinch Aluminum-free Baking Soda, divided
        (Bob's Redmill)
    ½ Acorn Squash, cooked and cut in 1 inch cubes or smaller
    7 cups purified Water, divided
    ½ cup chopped organic Onion
    1 tsp organic ground Cumin, or more to taste
    4 Tbsp. Braggs Liquid Amino Acids
    ½ cup each:
        chopped organic Carrots
        chopped organic Celery
        and any other chopped organic Vegetables of your
        choice (I like organic String Beans, Spinach, Swiss Chard,
        Carrots, Zucchini, Bok Choy, Chinese Cabbage, Leeks,
        Rutabagas, Jerusalem Artichokes).

Success Secret: If you want to eat more alkaline, goat milk products are alkaline whereas cow's milk products are acid. Also, if you can find a local goat dairy that really cares (check with your local health food store or the Internet), they may have these products that taste just like cow's milk, only much better!

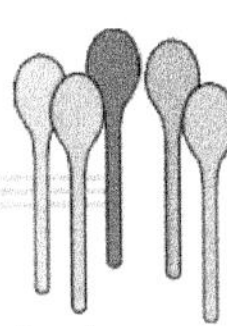

Vegans: Add slices of Avocado and sprouted organic Sunflower and Pumpkin Seeds as topping.

1. Soak Black Beans (Turtle Beans) in 3 cups Water with 1 tsp baking soda (to it make easier to digest). Soak for 24 hours, rinse after the first 12 hours. Rinse again after 12 more hours and just before cooking. You can refrigerate the soaked beans for a few days if you don't have time to cook them right away.

   Important Note: You may need to add more Water and Braggs Liquid Amino Acids as you add more veggies.

2. Mix and simmer on low for 2 hours: Soaked Beans, 4 cups Water, chopped Onion, Cumin, Braggs Liquid Amino Acids, I pinch Baking Soda (takes out the "wind") and Vegetables of choice.

3. Add cooked Squash. If you prefer a thicker soup base, simply blend a little of the soup and add it back in. Voila!

Success Secret: If you want great flavor in any of your culinary creations, just make sure to add enough good, healthy salt. Salt is a necessary ingredient for good health, but has a bad name due to the reaction people have to the processed kind that is laced with chemicals used to make it flow easily when it pours. Celtic Sea Salt or better yet, for absorption and flavor, pink Himalayan salt is full of minerals the body needs. Check with your doctor before making dietary changes.

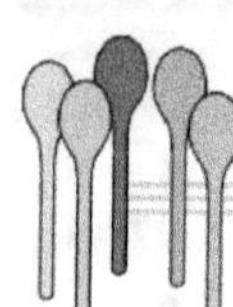
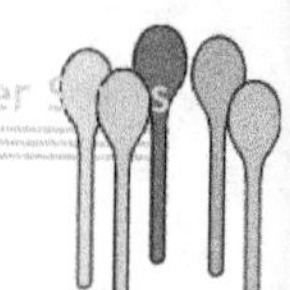

Variations

- If you like a smoother soup, blend it with soaked Almonds or Sprouted Grains such as Quinoa. Simply soak grains beforehand for about 4 hours.
- Add cooked Wild Rice (very low-glycemic and not really a grain) along with other Vegetables such as Celery and Onion. If you like other grains in the soup, soak them beforehand for about 4 hours and then cook in soup broth before adding meat back in, so meat doesn't get overdone and grains taste great.
- For more flavor, add a bit of organic Thyme, to taste (tastes like stuffing, yum!). Add thyme any time!

TRADITIONAL CHICKEN SOUP/STOCK

This is my Jewish mother's recipe. It took me awhile to get the measurements since she didn't measure unless baking and neither do I. I encourage you to taste what you are cooking in order to know what tastes best for you and your family.

Serves: Two to four people

Ingredients:

One whole small organic or free range Chicken
(for best flavor) with gizzards and all giblets removed
or 4 Chicken Breasts
Purified Water to cover Chicken in cooking pot
4 medium or 2 large organic Carrots
1 tsp or more Celtic Sea Salt, to taste
or 1 tsp or more Pink Himalayan Salt, to taste

1. Rinse Chicken with tap water and then rinse with purified Water. Place in pot and add Water to about two inches above Chicken. Bring to a boil on high heat; then turn down low until it just simmers.
2. While waiting for Water to boil, peel or wash Carrots well and slice in about 1-inch-thick slices.
3. Add Carrots and Salt to pot. Allow to simmer for at least one hour. Real Jewish chicken soup takes about eighteen hours, and the flavor is incredible, but who has time?
4. Lift out Chicken and remove meat from bones (if any) and chop. Taste Broth to see if it needs more Salt. You now have Soup Stock with which to work.
5. Use the stock as a base (and keep the chicken meat for another recipe, such as chicken salad) or you can return Chicken back to the pot with Vegetables of choice.

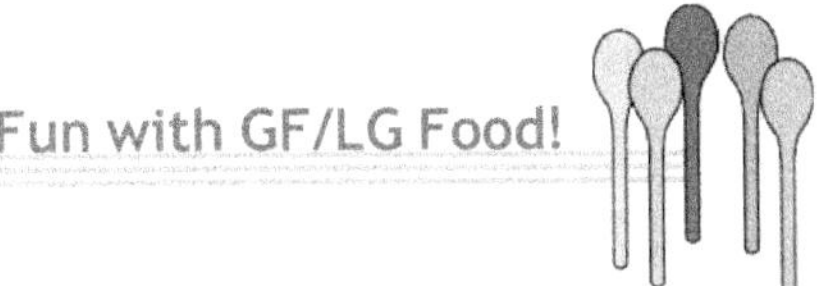

Variations

- Add 1 tsp freshly grated organic Lemon while cooking.
- For a uniquely full flavor, add ½ tsp organic Cumin.
- Add sautéed Mushrooms of choice.

Vegans: Use vegan soup broth and replace the milk with Savory Cashew Cream to taste. If unsure of amount, start with or ¼ cup.

Dairy-sensitive people: Replace milk with substitute of choice.

Nut-sensitive people: Add ¼ cup cooked Quinoa to blender for a creamier, milk-like look and taste.

CREAM OF ASPARAGUS SOUP

Yes, I know asparagus is expensive, but this is so yummy, it's worth it. And look at all the money you've saved on treats you can't buy! You deserve this.

Serves: Two to four people

Ingredients:

2 cups Chicken Stock
    or 1 Tbsp. Braggs Liquid Amino Acids to 1 cup Water
6-8 stalks of organic Asparagus
    or one package frozen organic Asparagus
1 small Carrot, peeled or scrubbed and sliced ¼ inch or so
    (unless using Chicken Stock that already has cooked carrots)
½ organic Onion, cut in small pieces
½ cup organic Milk (goat, cow, unsweetened almond)
    or ¼ cup organic dairy Cream
    or ¼ cup Savory Cashew Cream (p. 14, 15 or 40)

1. Bring soup stock to a boil.
2. While doing that, cut Onion, Asparagus and Carrots, if needed, and toss into soup stock.
3. When Vegetables are slightly tender (no need to cook until soft), take off heat, let cool and blend in blender.
4. When ready to serve, heat and add Milk or Cream of choice. You may garnish with very small dollop of Sour Cream and top with very slight sprinkle of Lemon Zest for flair.

Success Secret: When making cream soups, you can even use raw vegetables as long as your blender or food processor is able to cream them sufficiently.

Variations

- Add ¼ cup Quinoa right at the beginning before boiling Stock—it should be done by the time all Vegetables are added and cooked.
- Add ½ cup cooked Garbanzo Beans (lower in starch than other beans).

QUICK ITALIAN VEGETABLE SOUP

This is the real Italian way, mostly vegetables. The pasta and beans in minestrone are more of an Americanization.

Serves: Two to four people

Ingredients:

1 cup of your favorite organic Italian Red Sauce
(if you can't eat tomatoes, use ¼ cup Pesto and ¾ cup more Water)
2 cups purified Water with 2 Tbsp. Braggs Liquid Amino Acids or 2 cups Traditional Chicken Soup/Stock (p. 20)
½ cup fresh or frozen organic String Beans
¼ cup organic Onion, chopped
1 medium organic Carrot, sliced
2 large leaves of organic Swiss Chard, cut in small pieces
1 stalk organic Celery, sliced
½ medium organic Zucchini, quartered and sliced
½ tsp organic Fennel Seed, crushed
1 tsp organic Oregano
1 tsp organic Thyme
1 tsp organic Basil
¼ cup organic extra virgin, cold-pressed Olive Oil

1. Bring Water or Soup Stock to a boil along with the Italian Red Sauce.
2. While the stock is heating, slice Vegetables and add veggies, starting with Onion, String Beans and Carrot, then add Celery and Swiss chard, then Zucchini.
3. Cook just until Vegetables are tender, remove from stove, then add the Olive Oil.

Success Secret: To save time, slice and toss in the pot the harder vegetables first since they take longer to cook.

Variations

- Meat eaters may add cubed organic Beef and cook until Beef is done to make this a low-carb, better food-combining (no Potatoes) stew.
- Add organic Cabbage, Bok Choy or other light Vegetables for a different flavor and to stretch it. Also makes it a little less heavy.
- Add fresh organic Ginger for an Asian taste.
- Add organic Rosemary or Thyme for a savory flavor.

ROOT VEGETABLE STEW

This can be a main dish as well by adding browned beef or bison.

Serves: This recipe is measured in "per person" amounts.

Ingredients per person:
   1¼ heaping cups of veggies cut in ½-inch pieces:
      Rutabaga
      Parsnip
      Carrot
      Onion
      Celery
   1 cup purified Water
   2 Tbsp. Braggs Liquid Amino Acids
   ¼ tsp organic Rosemary

1. Place Vegetables in Water.
2. Add Braggs Liquid Amino Acids and Rosemary and simmer for 5 to 10 minutes or until done to your liking.
3. To thicken stew, blend half of stew until smooth or add ¼ cup per person cooked Quinoa or grind 1 Tbsp. per person Quinoa in clean or dedicated coffee grinder and cook into stew.

Success Secret: Success Secret: Experts in digestion say it takes 6 to 18 hours to digest meat, therefore it's best eaten at breakfast and lunch. I jokingly tell people I turn into a vegetarian after 3 p.m. (the opposite of a werewolf?) It has helped my energy to eat this way. Everyone is unique, so do what feels right to you and ask your own expert health practitioner.

Variations

- Garnish with chopped organic Veggies: Tomato, yellow Bell Pepper and Parsley, Cilantro, green Onion or Avocado.
- For a creamier taste add a dollop of organic Sour Cream or Savory Cashew Cream (p. 14, 15 or 40).
- Try it with any or all of the garnishes suited to your taste. I like to put a smorgasbord of ingredients on the table and see what people combine themselves. I get new food creation ideas that way, too!

Golden Chalice
CUCUMBER GAZPACHO

A light summer soup that is completely raw. It can be filled in to create a main meal for really hot days when you feel like eating lightly.

Serves: Two people

Ingredients:

　　1 cup (10 oz.) organic Cucumber
　　2 tsp fresh squeezed organic Lemon Juice
　　$\frac{1}{8}$ tsp Celtic Sea Salt, to taste
　　　　or $\frac{1}{8}$ tsp Pink Himalayan Salt, to taste
　　2 tsp Braggs Liquid Amino Acids
　　1 Tbsp. (½ oz) organic Onion
　　½ cup purified Water
　　Optional: ½ organic ripe Tomato

1. Cut up Cucumber in 1-inch or so slices.
2. Add remaining ingredients to blender or food processor, blend until smooth.
3. Pour into bowls.

> **Success Secret:** Be creative! Think of flavors you like and test them. Remember to test just a small amount, like a tablespoon or ¼ cup first, with your idea.

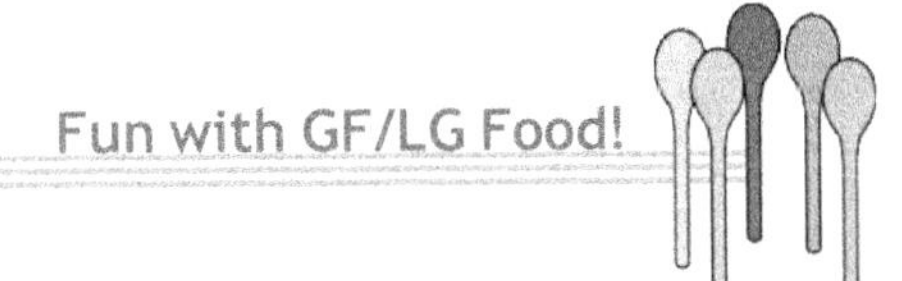

Chapter 3
Side Dishes, Salad Dressings, and Sauces

In this chapter, you'll find the secrets to a superb meal...the lovely, luscious, lingering tastes that accompany a fine meal. Soups quell that hard-earned hunger, salads tickle the palate, and sauces make everything sing with flavor, richness and life!

Recipes beginning with the words *"Golden Chalice"* are from my former gluten-free, diabetic-friendly restaurant of the same name.

Success Secret: Rather than steaming, I bake vegetables because then I don't lose any nutrients or flavor to the steam water, but if you do want to steam, you can use the water later for soup stock.

Variations

- Cut and peel Broccoli stems first, then slice in spears. Cook as you do the Asparagus.
- Cut Swiss Chard in small pieces, including stems. Cook as you do Asparagus, covering so it doesn't dry out. If the Chard isn't frozen, you may add 2 Tbsp. of purified Water to keep more moist.
- Peel Jerusalem Artichokes and cut in slices. Cook as you do Asparagus but longer. Check with a fork to see when done.
- Trim Green Beans and cook as you do Asparagus.
- Reader Shyrl Springer suggests adding mustard to Hollandaise Sauce for a new twist and to bring flavor up. She and her husband like it on Asparagus and modified Eggs Benedict.

Vegans: Replace Safflower Mayonnaise with Vegan Mayo (p. 38).

Side Dishes

ASPARAGUS WITH MOCK HOLLANDAISE SAUCE

A creamy, lemony sauce does not have to have flour or cream! I'm partial to buttery flavors myself, but with a lemon sauce and fresh, succulent asparagus, it's not even necessary, so if you can't eat dairy, no worries!

Serves: Two to four people

Ingredients:

½ lb fresh or frozen organic Asparagus
1 Tbsp. organic Ghee (clarified butter)
   or 1 Tbsp. Sunflower Oil
2 Tbsp. freshly squeezed organic Lemon Juice
¼ tsp Celtic Sea Salt
   or ¼ tsp Pink Himalayan Salt
2 Tbsp. purified Water
½ tsp Arrowroot Powder
   1 Tbsp. Hain Safflower Mayonnaise

1. Place cleaned fresh or frozen organic Asparagus stalks in covered oven-safe cookware and place in oven or toaster oven to bake at 350 °F for 5 minutes or until done to your liking. I like mine crisp and still bright green. If you prefer, you may steam or stir-fry them.
2. While Asparagus is cooking, blend together in small saucepan: Lemon Juice, Salt, Water and Arrow Root Powder. Heat on medium to high heat while stirring constantly until thick.
3. Stir in Ghee or Oil and Mayonnaise of choice and you're done! Refrigerate leftover.

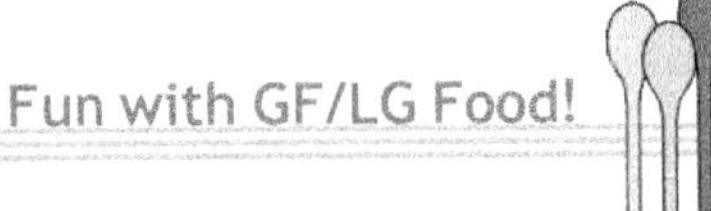

Variations

- Add any amount of other Vegetables to make this side dish lower glycemic-index. For example, add extra chopped Onions, chopped organic Cauliflower, chopped Carrots or any other Veggie of choice while cooking.
- Add one clove crushed organic Garlic for garlic lovers.
- Top with organic Sour Cream or Savory Cashew Cream (p. 14 or 40)
- Bacon Bits or other Smoked Meat or Meat-Substitutes may be added for texture and flavor.

Golden Chalice
BLACK BEAN SIDE DISH

This recipe can be easily adapted to either soup or side dish, depending on how thick you make it. The soup is very versatile and can be like chili as a main meal, too. The Black Bean and Squash Soup recipe (p. 15) is similar, but has a variety of other vegetables added, if you want to experiment with a more colorful side dish.

Serves: Two to four people

Ingredients:

1 cup Organic Black Beans (Turtle Beans)
1 tsp plus 1 pinch Aluminum-free Baking Soda, divided (Bob's Redmill)
5 cups purified Water, divided
$\frac{1}{3}$ cup chopped Organic Onion
1 tsp Organic Cumin
2 Tbsp. Braggs Liquid Amino Acids

1. Soak Black Beans in 3 cups purified Water with 1 tsp Baking Soda (to it make easier to digest). Soak for 24 hours, rinse after the first 12 hours, then rinse again after 12 more hours and again just before cooking. If necessary, you can refrigerate the soaked beans for a few days if you don't have time to cook them right away.
2. Simmer on low for 2 hours: 2 cups purified Water with soaked Beans, Onion, Cumin, Braggs Liquid Amino Acids, 1 pinch Baking Soda (takes out the "wind").
3. If Water is left over, boil without lid until it is thick enough.
4.

Success Secret: Using garlic sparingly allows other flavors to come through. Top chefs use it rarely. A side note for health: An obscure study showed garlic to be better used medicinally (how it's used traditionally in Europe) because it may tend to affect memory. This is not true for everyone, but I found my memory is better without eating garlic! I'm not a doctor, and we are all unique, so judge for yourself; I just know what works for me and you must discover that for yourself as well.

Variations

- Add 1-2 stalks organic Green Onion, chopped to your liking.
- Top with organic Sour Cream of choice or Savory Cashew Cream (p. 14 or 40).
- Top with organic Gravy of choice or see Gravy recipes p. 44 or 75).

Vegans: Use Oil instead of Ghee.

MASHED RUTABAGAS

A traditional family favorite for the holidays in some households, rutabagas have more flavor than potatoes and are lower in starch. Very warming winter food.

Serves: Four to six people

Ingredients:

2 medium organic Rutabagas
¼ cup Ghee
    or ¼ cup Sunflower
    or ¼ cup Safflower Oil
¼ cup organic Cream, Vegan Cream,
    or ¼ cup Savory Cashew Cream (p. 14 or 40)
1 tsp Celtic Sea Salt
    or 1 tsp Pink Himalayan Salt
¼ tsp organic pepper of choice

1. Peel, slice and steam Rutabagas until very soft and easy to mash (try against side of pot after 20 minutes).
2. Mash with fork or potato masher or food processor.
3. Add remaining ingredients and serve.

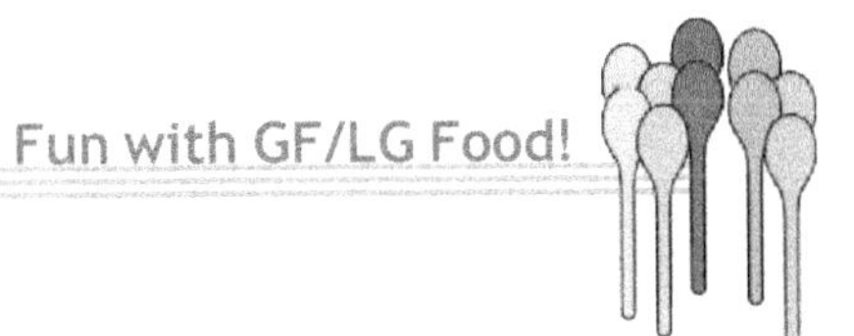

STRING BEANS WITH MUSHROOMS AND ONIONS

Traditional string bean side dish with French onions for the holidays is usually made with not-so-healthy ingredients. This dish is much better for you and very tasty, too!

Serves: Four to six people

Ingredients:
  1 lb frozen, French cut organic Green Beans
  1 cup organic Shitake Mushrooms
  1 cup organic White or Yellow Onion
  ½ tsp Celtic Sea Salt
      or ½ tsp Pink Himalayan Salt
  ¼ cup organic Ghee
      or ¼ cup high heat Sunflower Oil
  ¼ cup organic Cream
      or ¼ cup Savory Cashew Cream (p. 14 or 40)
      or ¼ cup alternative

1. Sauté Onions in Ghee or Oil until Onions are browned and even a little crisp, if you like them that way, then set aside.
2. Sauté Mushrooms until nearly cooked through.
3. Add frozen or thawed Green Beans and Salt. Sauté until done.
4. Blend in Cream of choice and top with browned Onion before serving warm in baking dish.

Side Salads and Dressings

Golden Chalice
FRESH GINGER-SESAME SALAD DRESSING

This dressing is great with toasted organic Sesame Seeds on the salad. To serve as a main meal, it goes well with marinated freshly grilled salmon, shrimp, chicken or beef on salad (see marinade and instructions for salad, p. 64) or sprouted organic almonds (soaked for 16 hours and rinsed twice).

Makes: About 1 cup
Ingredients:

    2 inches (or more, to your liking) organic Ginger Root,
        cut into chunks
    2 Tbsp. organic Lemon Juice
        or 2 Tbsp. organic Apple
        Cider or 2 Tbsp. Balsamic
        Vinegar
    ½ cup organic, cold-pressed Sesame Oil
    2 Tbsp. Braggs Liquid Amino Acids
    $1/8$ tsp Sweet Leaf Stevia
        or other form of Stevia, to taste
    1 Tbsp. Unsweetened Apple Sauce

1. Blend all ingredients until smooth. You're done!
2. Keep refrigerated.

Success Secret: Stevia is usually found as white powder or a clear liquid. The more natural kinds, which I'd recommend for ease on your body, are green powder, usually sold in bulk at health food stores, or the concentrated brown liquid. Use to taste.

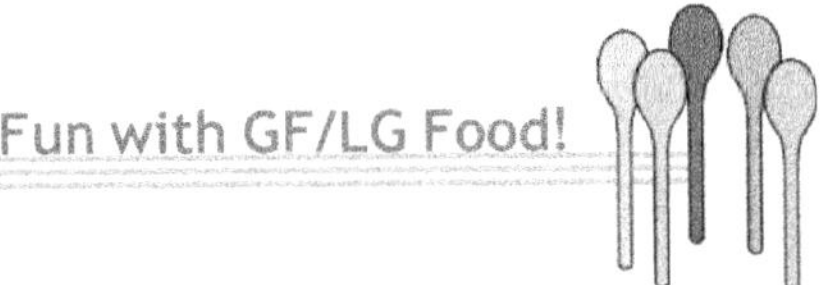

Variations

- Try different dressings, such as Yogurt, Sour Cream or the salad dressings in this chapter.
- Try different Herbs, particularly fresh Herbs like organic fresh Basil, Dill or Rosemary.
- Top with organic sprouted Seeds or Nuts of choice and any Meat or Fish for a quick lunch.

Vegans: Replace Safflower Mayonnaise with Vegan Mayo (p. 38).

NAPA CABBAGE SALAD

Serves: Four to six people

Ingredients:

1 cup chopped or grated organic Napa (Chinese) Cabbage
   or any Cabbage
¼ cup thinly sliced organic Celery
¼ cup diced organic Yellow and/or Red Bell Pepper
¼ cup shredded or chopped Organic Carrots
2 Tbsp. organic Hain Safflower Mayonnaise, or more
¼ tsp or more Pink Himalayan Salt
   or Celtic Sea Salt, to taste

1. Mix all ingredients together well and use or refrigerate for flavors to blend.

Success Secret: Green bell pepper is not as easy on the digestion as red and yellow, according to digestion experts. Also, all bell peppers are nightshades and should be eaten not-so-often according to health experts. I find I feel better then and the peppers and other nightshades become a treat. Other nightshade vegetables include potatoes (except for yams and sweet potatoes), eggplant, tomato and all other forms of pepper, both red and black. For a tangy, hot taste, try ginger root or wasabi or other kinds of mustard.

Vegans: Replace Safflower Mayonnaise with Vegan Mayo (p. 38).

Golden Chalice
LEMON-PESTO DRESSING

What to do with extra pesto? The following salad dressing is a big hit and quite simple to make: but don't limit yourself to salad! It tastes great on fish, chicken or stirred into rice or other grains

Makes: About 1 cup

Ingredients:
- ½ cup Hain Safflower Mayonnaise
    - or ½ cup homemade Safflower Mayonnaise
    - or ½ cup Savory Cashew Cream
- 2 tsp Organic Classic Pesto (p. 45 or 67)
- 2 tsp Organic Lemon Juice
- 2 Tbsp. Organic Cold Pressed Virgin Olive Oil

1. Mix in bowl or jar, then use immediately or refrigerate.

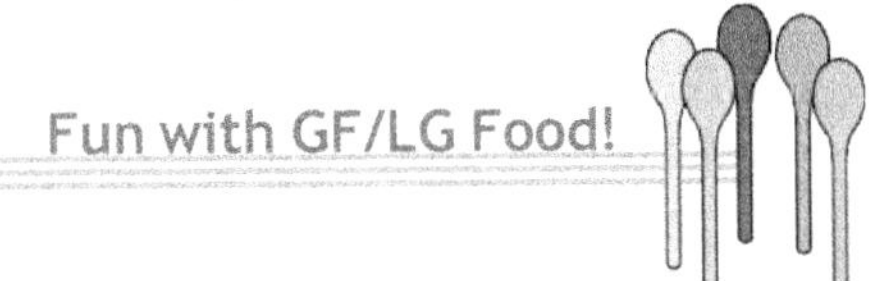

Vegans: Replace the Goat Milk with any Protein Substitute, such as soaked Nuts and Seeds and/or vegan Cheese of choice. Use one with a neutral flavor.

Golden Chalice GREEK SALAD

The Kalamata Olive Dressing below allows the flavor of the olives to permeate the whole salad.

Serves: Depends on size of salads you want and whether using for main dish

Ingredients (determine quantities for yourself):
Fresh organic Romaine Lettuce, washed
    and torn in bite-size bits
Fresh organic Tomato
Organic European Cucumber (easier to digest)
Feta Cheese from Goat Milk, if possible, crumbled
Organic Red Onion, thinly sliced
Fresh Mint Leaves, if available, cut in small, thin strips

1. Arrange all ingredients as you like, using your artistic eye to make it pretty!

Vegans: Replace Safflower Mayonnaise with Vegan Mayo (p. 38).

Golden Chalice KALAMATA OLIVE DRESSING

Very popular with some of our guests at *The Golden Chalice* they would come to eat there just for this dressing!

Makes: About 1 cup

Ingredients:
¾ cup *Golden Chalice* House Dressing (p. 34)
1 oz. chopped organic Kalamata Olives
2 oz. Hain Safflower Mayonnaise
¼ tsp Oregano

1. Put all ingredients in the blender and blend well.
2. Keep refrigerated until serving, or use right away.

Golden Chalice
HOUSE DRESSING

This dressing was the favorite at the *"Golden Chalice,"* second only to the Ginger-Sesame dressing.

Makes: About 1 cup

Ingredients:
¾ cup organic, cold-pressed virgin Olive Oil
2 Tbsp. Lemon Juice
1 Tbsp. Braggs Liquid Amino Acids
½ tsp dry, organic Oregano
　　crushed between fingers or in mortar and pestle
pinch Celtic Sea Salt
　　or pinch Pink Himalayan Salt

1. Place all ingredients in jar or blender and shake or blend. Use or refrigerate.

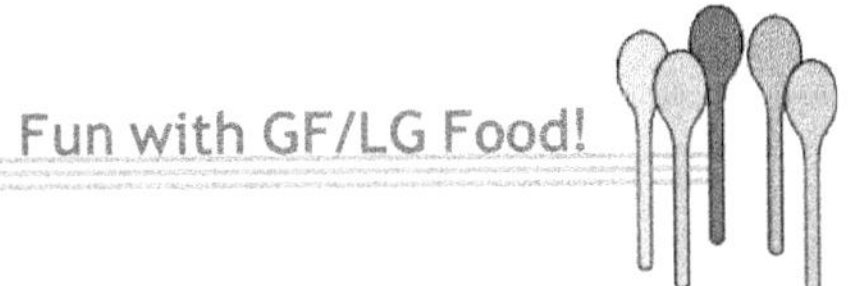

Variation

- Add ripe organic Avocado, sliced and arranged in circle around edge of salad. Or, make Guacamole (p. 9) and dot around edges of salad.

FIESTA SALAD

This can be a main meal by adding the side dish of black beans and/or meat or fish or your choice.

Serves: Depends on size of salads you want and if using for main dish.

Ingredients (determine quantities for yourself):
    Organic Field Greens
    Organic Red and Yellow Bell Peppers
    Fresh, ripe Organic Tomato
    Organic Red Onion
    Organic Kalamata or Black Olives
    Organic Goat Feta Cheese, grated
    Organic Black Beans, cooked (p. 27)
        Creamy Salsa Dressing (p. 36)
        Sprouted Soufflé Flatbread (p. 102)

1. Arrange Field Greens of your choice on each dinner or salad plate.
2. Top with sliced or chopped: Bell Peppers, Tomato, Onion, Olives, Cheese. Then top with Black Beans.
3. Serve with Creamy Salsa Dressing, and if you like, Sprouted Soufflé Flatbread—reminds me of cornbread but has a much lower-glycemic level and is much better for making this meal a complete protein.

Vegans: Replace Safflower Mayonnaise with Vegan Mayo (p. 38).

CREAMY SALSA DRESSING

You can easily adjust this to different members of the family by making it mild, then putting their favorite high-temperature salsa in front of the "hot shots."

Makes: About $1^3/_4$ cups

Ingredients:
    1 cup Hain Safflower Mayonnaise
    ¼ cup Salsa (mild to hot — depending on your preference)
    Celtic Sea Salt, to taste
       or Pink Himalayan Salt, to taste

1. Stir together and you're done!

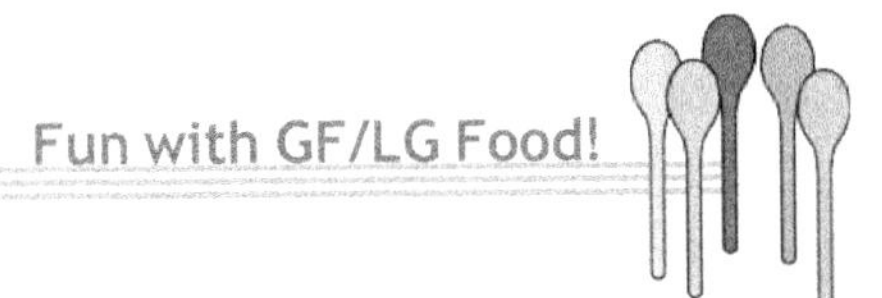

Golden Chalice
SWEET WASABI DRESSING

This dressing goes well with Ahi Tuna Salad (p. 72).

Makes: About ½ cup

Ingredients:

> 1 Tbsp. Unsweetened Apple Sauce
> 1¼ tsp Wasabi powder (green Mustard served with Sushi)
> ¼ cup organic, cold-pressed Sesame Oil
> 2 tsp Braggs Liquid Amino Acids
> ¼ tsp Sweet Leaf Stevia
>   or other form of Stevia, to taste

1. Blend all ingredients in blender except for Stevia. Taste before adding to insure it will not be too sweet for your taste.

Variations

- Add 1 tsp fresh, organic Rosemary leaves, finely chopped.
- Add 1 tsp of your favorite Pesto (p. 45).
- Add your favorite Hot Peppers, dry ground, or finely chopped fresh.

Sauces

Some of these may be repeated in the book, but here you have all necessary sauce or condiment alternatives in one place.

Golden Chalice
VEGAN MAYO

Makes: About $1/3$ cup

Ingredients:

¼ cup Savory Cashew Cream (p. 14, 15 or 40)
1 tsp organic Lemon Juice
$1/8$ tsp Celtic Sea Salt
    or $1/8$ tsp Pink Himalayan Salt
$1/8$ tsp organic Dry Mustard
½ tsp Unsweetened Apple Sauce

1. Mix ingredients together until well-incorporated.
2. Use within two days.

Success Secret: Be creative! For vegan mayo or other vegan dishes, find flavors you love to overtake the non-traditional flavors that make the base, like the cashews that replace the normal egg base.

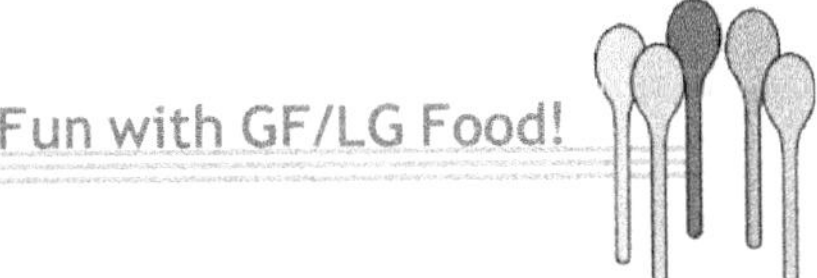

Variation

* Reader Shyrl Springer suggests adding Mustard to Hollandaise Sauce to give it a little more flavor and color, but use yellow Mustard Powder to be sure of no sugar, white vinegar or gluten. She and her husband like it on Asparagus and modified Eggs Benedict.

Vegans: Replace Safflower Mayonnaise with Vegan Mayo (p. 38).

MOCK HOLLANDAISE SAUCE

A creamy, lemony sauce does not have to have flour or cream! I'm partial to buttery flavors myself, but with a lemon sauce and fresh, succulent veggies, even if you can't eat dairy, no worries! The flavor will still be great. Also, you can get natural, organic butter flavor at your local health food store.

Serves: Two to four people

Ingredients:
- 1 Tbsp. organic Ghee (clarified butter) or 1 Tbsp. Sunflower Oil
- 2 Tbsp. freshly squeezed organic Lemon Juice
- ¼ tsp Celtic Sea Salt or ¼ tsp Pink Himalayan Salt
- 2 Tbsp. purified Water
- ½ tsp Arrowroot Powder (thickeners) 1 Tbsp. Hain Safflower Mayonnaise

1. Blend together in small Saucepan: Lemon Juice, Salt, Water and Arrowroot Powder. Heat on medium to high heat while stirring constantly until thick.
2. Stir in Ghee or Oil and Mayonnaise of choice and you're done! Use or refrigerate.

Variation

- Simply add any herbs, Spices or condiments you like, ¼ tsp to start, then taste as you add small amounts more to make it to your liking.

Golden Chalice
SAVORY CASHEW CREAM (Vegan)

When you need cream without sweeteners, dairy or soy, here's a raw food alternative.

Makes: About ¾ cup

Ingredients:

- ½ cup organic Cashews, germinated
  (soaked for eight hours and rinsed well, becomes ²/₃ cup after soaking—use within two days, rinse daily)
- ¼ cup or more purified Water, depending on preference
- 2 dashes Celtic Sea Salt
  or 2 dashes Pink Himalayan Salt

1. Soak Cashews for four more hours in purified Water and rinse well.
2. Blend all ingredients in blender or food processor until smooth.
3. Refrigerate or use immediately. Freeze unused portion within 2 days.

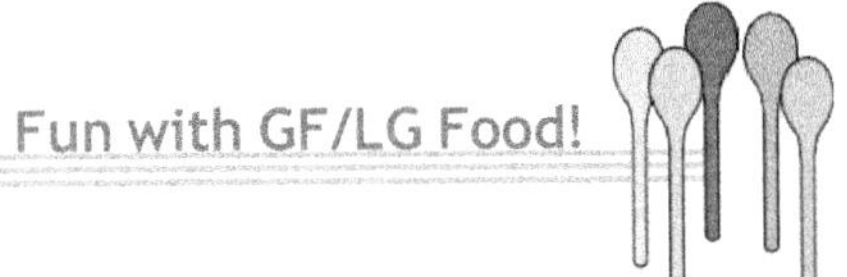

Variation

- Add any flavor or extract of your choice from Lemon Zest and Orange Zest to Coconut or coffee flavor. Play around with organic gluten-free flavorings and have fun!

Nut-sensitive people: In place of organic cream or Sweet Cashew Cream in any recipe, try Coconut Milk, found in health food and Asian stores. Use the creamy part which has risen to the top of the can. You can flavor and sweeten it to taste the same way you would Sweet Cashew Cream.

Golden Chalice
SWEET CASHEW CREAM (Vegan)

For those who like a smooth, creamy alternative to dairy creams.

Makes: About ¾ cup

Ingredients:
 ½ cup organic Cashews, germinated
  (soaked for eight hours and rinsed well—becomes ²/₃ cup after soaking—use within two days, rinse daily)
 ¼ cup purified Water
 2 dashes Celtic Sea Salt
  or 2 dashes Pink Himalayan Salt
 1 tsp organic Vanilla Extract
  or 1 tsp Vanilla Flavor (Celiacs may not tolerate extract)
 1 Tbsp. organic pure Maple Syrup
  or ¼ cup Unsweetened Apple Sauce
 ½ tsp Sweet Leaf Stevia
  or other form of Stevia, to taste

1. Soak Cashews for four more hours in purified Water and rinse well.
2. Blend all ingredients in blender or food processor until smooth.
3. Refrigerate or use immediately. Freeze unused portion within 2 days.

Variations

- Use 1½ to 2 cups fruit of choice—Blueberries, Strawberries, Mango, etc.—in place of Bananas, or use 1 cup each Bananas and other Fruit. Combine whatever Fruits you like.
- This sauce is fairly thin, as I like my sauce to seep into my pancakes. To thicken your sauce simply blend 1 Tbsp. Arrowroot into the Water first, then stir constantly until thickened.

Wheat and gluten-sensitive people: Gluten-free vanilla extract is now available in some health food stores and online.

BANANA-ORANGE SAUCE

Very versatile, you can make this into any kind of fruit sauce you wish.

Makes: About 2½ cups

Ingredients:
- ¼ cup organic Ghee (clarified butter)
- 3 small to medium, ripe organic Bananas
- ½ cup Unsweetened Apple Sauce
- 1 cup or more purified Water
- 1 tsp organic Vanilla Extract
  - or 1 tsp vanilla Flavoring for Celiacs
- ½ tsp organic Orange Extract
  - or Grated Peel of 1 organic Orange
- ½ tsp Celtic Sea Salt
  - or ½ tsp Pink Himalayan Salt
- ¼ tsp Stevia (or other form of Stevia, to taste)
  - **and** either Unsweetened Apple Sauce or organic Maple Syrup, to taste

1. Melt Ghee in medium-size saucepan.
2. Cut up Bananas; add them and Unsweetened Apple Sauce to hot Ghee, sauté for about 1 minute.
3. Add Water, Extracts, Salt, Stevia and Unsweetened Apple Sauce or Maple Syrup if you like. Do taste and use your own sweetness meter!
4. Simmer for 5 minutes, then serve hot.
5. Refrigerate to store leftovers. (Ha! 'Doubt there will be any.)

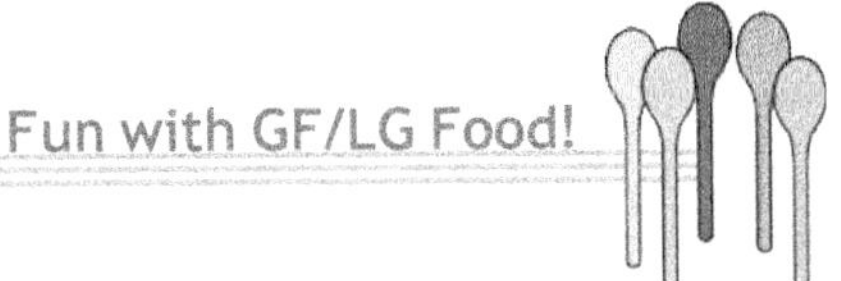

Variations

- Add ½ cup organic Shitake Mushrooms, sautéed.
- Add ½ cup organic chopped Onions, sautéed.
- Add 1 clove crushed organic Garlic, sautéed.
- Add 1 tsp organic Sage and Thyme to make it taste like stuffing!

Vegans: Replace drippings with Braggs Liquid Amino Acids.

QUICK GRAVY

For vegans or meat-eaters. Can be used with meat, potatoes, stuffing, veggies, grains—whatever!

Makes: One cup—multiply as needed

Ingredients:

1 cup Meat Drippings,
  or 1 cup Broth
  or 1 cup Braggs Liquid Amino Acids if no drippings/broth available
1 tsp Arrowroot Powder to thicken (find at health food store)
½ tsp Celtic Sea Salt
  or ½ tsp Pink Himalayan Salt
Organic White Peeper
  or Black Pepper, to taste

1. Stir Salt into liquid, then Arrowroot Powder into cool or just warm liquid (not hot).
2. Bring to a simmer, stirring constantly. Remove from heat as soon as it is thick enough for you. If you want it thicker, mix separately more Arrowroot Powder with just enough Water to melt, then add to liquid on stove and heat and stir once more until thick enough.
3. Add Pepper last, and do not cook it as it can be hard on intestines when heated.

Success Secret: Pepper is best for digestive system when not cooked otherwise it can be an irritant.

Vegans and dairy-sensitive people: Replace Parmesan Cheese with vegan Cheese or simply use added Salt—½ tsp Celtic Sea Salt or ½ tsp Pink Himalayan Salt.

CLASSIC PESTO

Makes: About 1 cup

Ingredients:
I cup loosely packed fresh, washed organic Basil Leaves
¼ cup Pine Nuts
¼ cup shredded organic Parmesan Cheese
¼ cup organic cold-pressed, virgin Olive Oil

1. Blend in blender

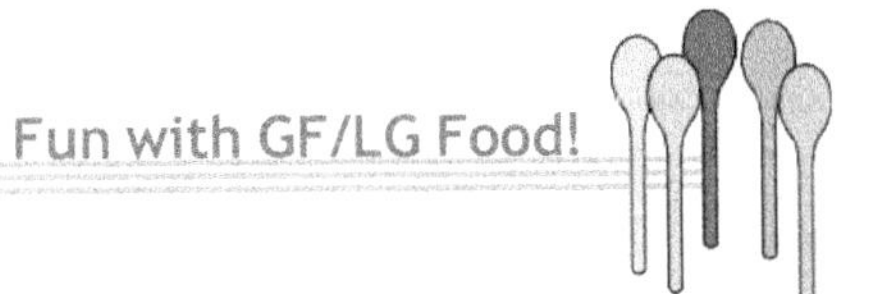

SPECIAL SAUCE

The "Special Sauce" they use in most fast food restaurants is so simple it's unbelievable. This is how I think it's done and how it tastes right to me. Here you go:

Makes: About $^2/_3$ cup

Ingredients (adjust to your personal taste):
   ¼ cup organic Ketchup or
      1 Tbsp. Tomato Paste, to avoid any sweeteners
   ½ cup Hain Safflower Mayonnaise
   1 tsp Celtic Sea Salt
      or 1 tsp Pink Himalayan Salt

1. Stir together all ingredients and taste. Add whatever you like to make it taste the way you want.

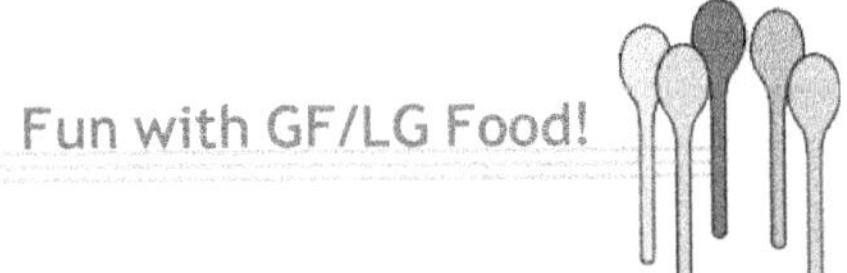

Chapter 4
Main Dishes

So many things to eat are loaded with sugar, starch and gluten...but have no fear, the GF/LG Cook is here! Enjoy some of your favorite comfort foods with style, flavor and most important...love!

Recipes beginning with the words *"Golden Chalice"* are from my former gluten-free, diabetic-friendly restaurant of the same name.

Variations

- Chop organic fresh Tomato and sprinkle on top of Sauce after putting it all together.
- Chop organic fresh Red Bell Pepper and sprinkle on top of Sauce after putting it all together.
- If you prefer scrambled Eggs or omelets, replace poached Eggs with them.

Vegans: Replace Eggs with vegan Protein of choice. Place on top of spinach.

Dairy-sensitive people: Replace Ghee with Olive Oil.

Breakfast or Brunch

EGGS BENEDICT FLORENTINE

A very filling breakfast, you'll win hearts with this one! And you don't have to use poached eggs if you don't like them. You're the Boss!

Serves: Two to four people

Ingredients:

½ lb fresh or frozen organic Spinach
    If frozen, squeeze out Water
Mock Hollandaise Sauce
2 Eggs per person
2 pieces of Sprouted Soufflé Flatbread (p. 102) per person
1 Tbsp. Ghee or Olive Oil per person
    or any amount for personal choice

1. Make mock Hollandaise Sauce.
2. Steam or bake Spinach and keep warm, or time it so it's done when the Eggs and toast are done. You have to be really fast to do all this together or have some help!
3. Poach Eggs. While poaching Eggs, toast Bread and spread with organic Ghee.
4. Cover Bread with light layer of Spinach.
5. Place Eggs on top, then cover with Sauce and serve immediately.

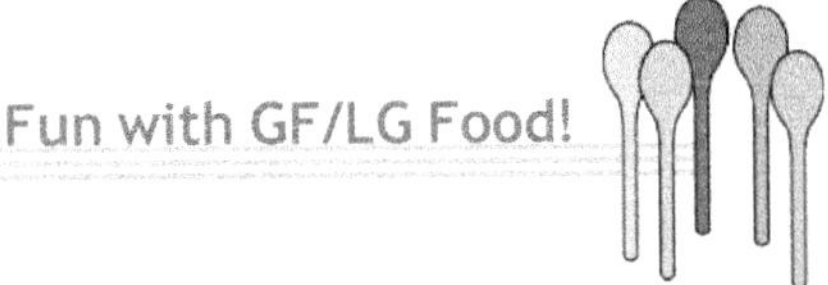

Variation

- Reader Shyrl Springer suggests adding mustard to Hollandaise Sauce for a new twist and to bring flavor up. She and her husband like it on Asparagus and modified Eggs Benedict.

Vegans: Replace Safflower Mayonnaise with Vegan Mayo (p. 38).

MOCK HOLLANDAISE SAUCE

A creamy, lemony sauce does not have to have flour or cream! I'm partial to buttery flavors myself, but with a lemon sauce and fresh, succulent veggies, even if you can't eat dairy, no worries! The flavor will still be great. Also, you can get natural, organic butter flavor at your local health food store.

Serves: Two to four people

Ingredients:

- 1 Tbsp. organic Ghee (clarified butter)
    - or 1 Tbsp. Sunflower Oil
- 2 Tbsp. freshly squeezed organic Lemon Juice
- ¼ tsp Celtic Sea Salt
    - or ¼ tsp Pink Himalayan Salt
- 2 Tbsp. pure Water
- ½ tsp Arrowroot Powder
    - 1 Tbsp. Hain Safflower Mayonnaise

1. Blend together in small saucepan: Lemon Juice, Salt, Water and Arrowroot Powder. Heat on medium to high heat, stirring constantly until thick.
2. Stir in Ghee or Oil and Mayonnaise of choice and you're done! Use or refrigerate.

Variations

- Sprinkle ½ tsp dry organic Dill Weed on top of Omelet. Makes nice presentation if you don't have veggies on top, and the flavor is wonderful for some combinations. The secret to full Dill flavor is not cooking it.
- Toss ½ tsp dry, crushed organic Rosemary leaves or 1 tsp fresh into blender along with Eggs.

FLUFFY OMELET

Omelets make wonderful main dishes almost anytime. See Frittata recipe in lunch and dinner recipes (p. 74).

Serves: This recipe is measured in "per person" amounts.

Ingredients per person:

　　2 organic Eggs
　　½ tsp Celtic Sea Salt
　　　　or ½ tsp Pink Himalayan Salt
　　1 Tbsp. purified Water
　　 Dash of Pepper (optional)
　　2 Tbsp. Ghee,
　　　　or 2 Tbsp. Bacon Grease
　　　　or 2 Tbsp. Oil of Choice, which can withstand high heat
　　½ cup organic Vegetables of choice
　　2 Tbsp. organic Goat Feta
　　　　or 2 Tbsp. Chevre (Goat) Cheese, any flavor you
　　　　　　like (herb, garlic, rosemary, etc.)

Success Secret: For more flavor when using dried Herbs; crush first between fingers or in mortar and pestle or in dedicated coffee grinder. Careful of using fingers when the dried herbs have sharp edges or points, like Rosemary.

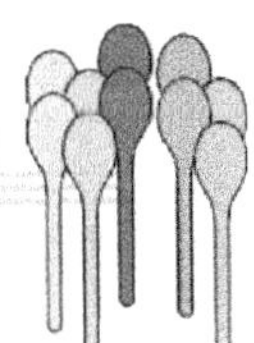

Important Note: Yes, bacon grease is a high-heat cooking oil! And yes, I eat organic bacon and save the grease in a jar in the fridge. (Hey we don't have a lot of other perks, so we get to have some fun with our food—unless of course, your doctor says no...though my doctor says my HDLs and LDLs and all the Ls are the best he's ever seen—you do the math.)

1. Grate Feta or spoon out Chevre, ready to slap onto Omelet.
2. Chop your Vegetables in small pieces and sauté in Ghee or high-heat Oil, starting with Onions (let them get a little soft) and ending with Veggies that cook faster, like Zucchini or Tomatoes. Mushrooms absorb lots of Oil, so add more Oil if needed. I like using Bacon Grease.
3. Place first four Ingredients in blender, heat pan to medium with Ghee or Oil and while pan is heating, blend well.
4. Pour Omelet mix into pan and let cook until edges look done, then put Cheese on it, fold it and turn as best you can. I'm pretty inept at it (why I hired great line cooks) but I did have a knack for turning them at home after I cut them in half. My secret's out...you can use it too. Also, I like to make sure my Eggs are cooked through, so I turn the Omelet first (after cutting in as many pieces as I need to!) and then I put the Cheese on.
5. Pour on warm Veggies and serve with a flourish!

Success Secrets: The secret to a fluffy omelet is so simple it's ridiculous. Just blend the heck out of the eggs just before pouring into pan! Also, use water, not milk. Surprise!

Don't worry if you can't make a perfect looking omelet. Neither can I, so the veggies on top hide the fact that I've ruined the omelet by cutting it into pieces, however, it tastes great and no one that I've ever served cares.

Variations

- Substitute Zucchini and Carrots for Parsnips. Onion is optional.
- Substitute Zucchini and Carrots for Rutabaga. Onion is optional.
- Carrots: Substitute Zucchini for Carrots. Onion is optional.
- Simply toss in 1 Tbsp. fresh or 1 tsp dried organic Rosemary leaves (if dried, crush first in mortar and pestle or in dedicated coffee grinder)

VEGGIE "HASH BROWNS"

Hash browned potatoes used to be one of my favorite breakfast foods, so I found a low-glycemic alternative. And it's actually easier and quicker! Also, some of you may not be able to eat very many nightshades, so here are root vegetable potato alternatives:

Serves: Two to four people

Ingredients:
- ½ medium organic red Onion
- 1 medium organic Carrot
- 2 small organic Zucchinis
- 2 Tbsp. Ghee
  - or 2 Tbsp. organic high-heat Oil
  - (Grapeseed or high-heat Sunflower)

1. Thinly slice or julienne all Vegetables, Onion first, Carrot second and Zucchini third.
2. While slicing or using food processor, begin sauté of Onion, then toss in Carrots and last, Zucchini, as it needs the least cooking time.
3. Brown to your heart's content! Serve hot and fresh, but will easily keep to warm later.

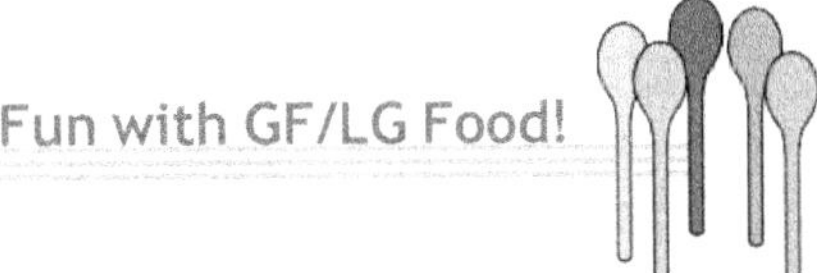

Variations

- Add ½ tsp organic Black or Red crushed Pepper ONLY if everyone's intestines are strong. This is an irritant when cooked. Or you can add when eating.
- Add any shredded Vegetables you like to stretch it and "hide your vegetables." I'd recommend Carrots, Zucchini or Cabbage.

TURKEY BREAKFAST SAUSAGE (or substitute meat/vegan meat)

To be sure of the healthiest Ingredients, you can make your own sausage more easily than you think! And the fresh flavor is so good.

Serves: Four to eight people

Ingredients:

1 lb. organic or free-range ground Turkey
   (dark meat is best)
2 Tbsp. Braggs Liquid Amino Acids
1 tsp Celtic Sea Salt
   or 1 tsp Pink Himalayan Salt
2 Tbsp. ground organic Sage
2 Tbsp. or more, to coat pan, Oil of Choice
   or 2 Tbsp. or more nitrite-free Bacon Grease

1. Mix all Ingredients in medium size bowl.
2. Heat organic Oil of Choice or nitrite-free Bacon Grease in fry pan at medium-high temperature.
3. Form Meat into patties and brown, then turn down heat to cook through until done. Test by cutting one open to see if done (sorry, but this is the best method I know, low-tech as it is, since juices don't flow too much from Turkey).

Success Secret: Smaller Bananas and smaller Zucchinis, as well as some other Fruits and Vegetables may be more flavorful. Use your intuition on that one. It works well for me most of the time.

Vegans: Replace Eggs with a combination of Protein Powder, soaked Cashews or Almond Meal, plus a small amount of Water and Egg Substitute of your choice.

Or, instead of Egg Substitute you may add 1 tsp or more Arrowroot Powder, according to how firm you like your pancakes.

Use Oil of Choice or virgin Coconut Oil to fry pancakes. Making these pancakes very small works best.

LOW-CARB PANCAKES or CRÊPES

This recipe is also in the dessert chapter—same one, so you can think of it for dessert as well, particularly in the form of crêpes. I learned from a French Canadian friend how to make the crêpes. You really can't go wrong as long as you have a well-greased or naturally non-stick pan. The consistency is very thin, but you can make it thicker, if you wish, for heavier crêpes, by simply adding more flour.

Serves: Eight to ten people

Ingredients:

Pancakes
    1 cup organic Cottage Cheese
        or 1 cup Ricotta Cheese
    6 organic or free-range Eggs
    ½ cup Amaranth
        or ½ cup Quinoa Flour
    ½ tsp Celtic Sea Salt
        or ½ tsp Pink Himalayan Salt
    I tsp aluminum-free Baking Powder (health food store)
    I tsp organic Vanilla Extract
        or I tsp Vanilla Flavor (Celiacs may not tolerate extract)
    ½ cup Ghee, Butter
        or ½ cup Oil of Choice
        or ½ cup virgin Coconut Oil
    I Tbsp. Lemon Peel
        (If mix is too liquid, add soaked Cashews to firm up)
    Ghee (clarified Butter) or Coconut Oil for frying

1. Blend all Ingredients in blender.
2. Optional, but recommended, for extra layers of flavor, add 1 tsp organic Cinnamon and ¼ tsp organic Almond Extract or Flavor.
3. Fry as you normally would pancakes or crêpes, using plenty of delicious oils like Ghee (clarified Butter) or Coconut Oil. Flip after bubbles burst, they will likely be done when the outside is brown.

Vegans and dairy-sensitive people: Replace Cheese with 1 cup soaked, germinated organic Cashews (soak raw Cashews in pure Water for four hours). Use ¼ cup Coconut Oil in place of Butter.

Crêpes

Same ingredients as pancakes, plus ¼ cup of purified Water (or more). Use toppings of your choice.

1. Follow directions for pancakes, but add ¼ cup Water or more to blender, depending on the thickness you'd like for the Crêpes.
2. Test a small one first. Make sure your pan is well greased unless it is non-stick (not recommended unless titanium, for health reasons—see p. 120)
3. Spread on pan with a large spoon, unless you are an expert crêpe-maker.
4. Top with pure organic maple syrup (for low-glycemic choice, Banana-Orange Sauce (p. 56, 43 or 83,) or other fruit Sauce variation.

Success Secret: Grind your own flours, seeds and herbs in a dedicated coffee grinder (not used for coffee). With my recipes, you use so little flour that you can grind it easily and quickly for freshness. You can make instant cereal that way, too!

Variations

- Use 1½ to 2 cups
  of any Fruit of choice—
  Blueberries,
  Strawberries, Mango,
  etc.—in place of
  Bananas, or 1 cup each
  Bananas and other Fruit.
  Combine whatever Fruits
  you like.
- This sauce is fairly thin,
  as I like my sauce to
  seep into my pancakes.
  To thicken your sauce
  simply blend 1 Tbsp.
  Arrowroot into the
  Water first, then stir
  constantly until
  thickened.

BANANA-ORANGE SAUCE

Very versatile, you can make this into any kind of fruit sauce
you wish.

Makes: About 2 ½ cups
Ingredients:

- ¼ cup organic Ghee (clarified butter)
- 3 small to medium, ripe organic Bananas
- ½ cup organic Unsweetened Apple Sauce
- 1 cup or more pure Water
- 1 tsp organic Vanilla Extract
    or 1 tsp Vanilla Flavor (Celiacs may not tolerate extract)
- ½ tsp organic Orange Extract
    or grated Peel of 1 organic Orange
- ½ tsp Celtic Sea Salt
    or ½ tsp Pink Himalayan Salt
- ¼ tsp Sweet Leaf Stevia
    or other form of Stevia, to taste
    and either Unsweetened Apple Sauce or organic Maple Syrup,
    to taste

1. Melt Ghee in medium-size saucepan.
2. Cut up Bananas; add them to hot Ghee, sauté for
   about one minute.
3. Add Water, Extracts, Salt, Stevia and Unsweetened
   Apple Sauce or Maple Syrup if you like. Do taste
   and use your own sweetness meter!
4. Simmer for 5 minutes, then serve hot.
5. Refrigerate leftovers. (Ha! Doubt there will be any.)

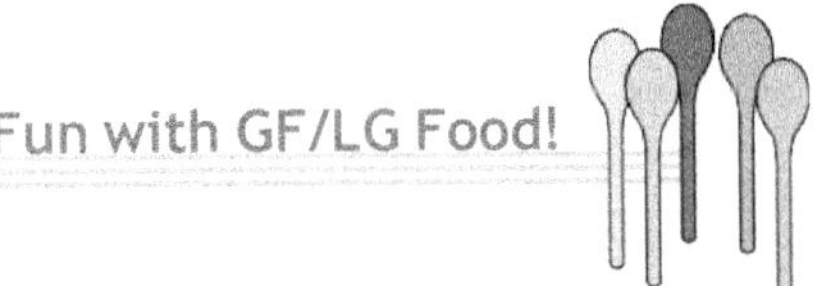

Variations

- After toasting Bread, spread with Ghee or Oil of Choice and sprinkle with freshly ground Cinnamon (ground in dedicated coffee grinder, not used for coffee).
- After toasting Bread, spread with Coconut Oil or Coconut Butter and sprinkle with finely ground unsweetened organic Coconut. Grind in dedicated coffee grinder (not used for coffee).
- After toasting Bread, sprinkle with Cinnamon (optional) then spread Almond Butter and slice Bananas on top (also optional). Cover with another piece of Bread and you can eat it on the run!

QUICK FRENCH TOAST

French toast can be a delightful, high protein meal if you use the high protein Sprouted Soufflé Flatbread. This bread is high in eggs already and very flavorful, so you can use it easily.

Serves: This recipe is measured in "per person" amounts.

Ingredients per person:
2 slices of Sprouted Soufflé Flatbread (p. 102)
Butter, to taste
Your favorite topping, to taste

1. Pop the Flatbread in the toaster or oven to heat, then Butter and pour on your favorite topping (see recipe for Banana-Orange Sauce, p. 56, 43 or 83, and variations or recipe for Cherry-Almond tart filling, p. 84), using whatever fruit you like. Enjoy!

Nut-sensitive people:
Replace Nut Meals with 1 cup Amaranth Flour and use extra Oil—¼ cup or more if needed to stick together.

Lunch or Dinner

Rosemary-Onion-Veggie Quiche for Everyone! (With dairy-free alternatives)

Makes: 1 pie, enough for three to four people

Ingredients:

Gluten-Free Crust
>   ¼ cup Amaranth or Quinoa Flour
>   ¾ cup Almond Meal Flour
>   2 Tbsp. Ghee or Oil of Choice
>   ½ tsp Himalyan or Celtic Sea Salt
>   ½ tsp Rosemary, finely ground
>   1 Egg or Egg Replacer (add 1 Tbsp. Protein Powder if using Egg Replacer)

1. Melt Ghee or Oil of Choice on low heat in pie pan, if you want to wash fewer pans.
2. Mix in Almond Meal and Flour, Salt and Egg or Egg Replacer with Protein Powder, if you use it, right in pie pan.

    Important Note: mix until mixture clumps together, so the Oil spreads evenly and will press well into pan and stay more firm.
3. Press into pie pan.

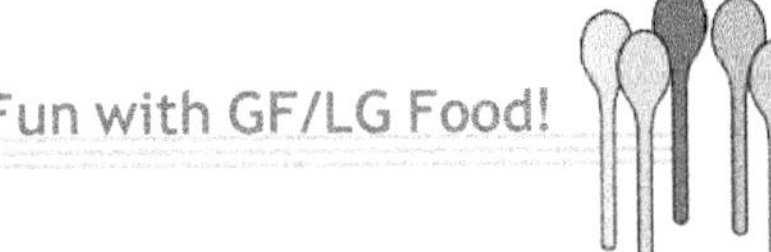

Vegans and dairy-sensitive people: Replace Goat Cheese with 1 cup soaked raw Cashews*. **Nut-sensitive people:** Use soaked sunflower seeds.

*You can keep soaked Cashews refrigerated in water up to two days after soaking. Then you must use or freeze them.

Filling

1 Tbsp. organic Ghee or Oil of Choice

½ cup Onion

¼ cup Leek

8 oz chopped chopped Veggies of Choice,
    I recommend zucchini, carrot, spinach, and/or chard

1 cup Water

1 cup organic Goat Cheddar
    or 1 cup Goat Feta Cheese,
    or fav. Cheese Substitute

3 organic Eggs
    or Egg Replacer to equal

1 tsp Braggs Liquid Amino Acids
    or 1 tsp Celtic Sea Salt
    or 1 tsp Pink Himalayan Salt

1 tsp Rosemary, chopped fresh or finely ground
    (use a dedicated coffee grinder, if needed)

1. Preheat oven to 350 °F.
2. Make crust in pan.
3. Slice Onion and Leek thinly and sauté in Ghee.
    When halfway done, add Veggies.
4. Line crust with Veggies.
5. Put rest of ingredients into blender or food processor.
6. Pour Egg mixture over Vegetables.
7. Bake at 350 °F for 30-40 minutes. Insert toothpick—it comes out clean when done.

Vegans: Replace Meat with Veggie Bacon of choice. Replace Safflower Mayonnaise with Vegan Mayo (p. 38).

BACON, LETTUCE and TOMATO SALAD

Smile if you love BLTs. Now you can have them in a much flavorful form that won't fall apart on you, because it already is apart and you eat it with a fork!

Serves: This recipe is measured in "per person" amounts.

Ingredients per person:
2 thick or 4 thin strips organic Bacon or Turkey Bacon
½ small to medium ripe Tomato
Organic Salad Greens
Hain Safflower Mayonnaise, to taste

1. Fry Bacon to your preferred crispness, or bake in oven and crumble or cut into pieces.
2. Arrange Salad Greens on plate and drop dollops of Mayonnaise (size dollops according to your love of Mayo) all over the salad. I like to then mix it up a bit to coat the Lettuce with Mayonnaise so its flavor is incorporated into the whole salad.
3. Cut Tomatoes into small pieces and decorate Salad Greens with Bacon and Tomato slices. Savor the flavor!

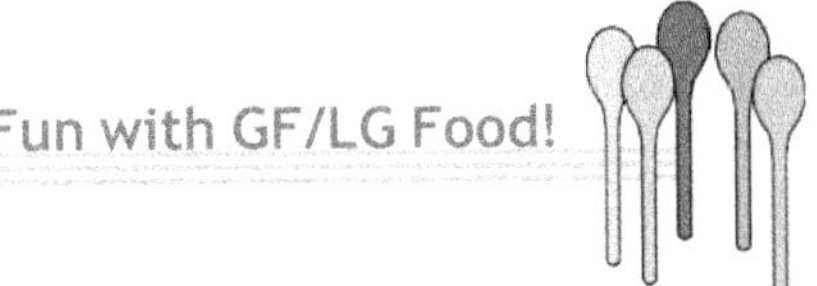

Variations

- Use soaked, germinated Sunflower Seeds instead of toasted, for more nutrients.
- Add 1 Tsp to 1 Tbsp. sliced or chopped organic Black Olives.
- Add chopped organic Tomato.

Vegans: Replace Eggs with Veggie Protein of choice, including Sunflower and Pumpkin Seeds that have been germinated and chopped.

Golden Chalice
EGG SALAD IN A BOAT

Lettuce wraps or Napa (Chinese) cabbage leaves work great with this simple classic with a twist.

Serves: This recipe is measured in "per person" amounts.

Ingredients per person:

2 organic Eggs
½ stalk organic Celery, chopped
2 Tbsp. organic toasted Sunflower Seeds (p. 12)
¼ tsp Celtic Sea Salt
   or ¼ tsp Pink Himalayan Salt
1 Tbsp. Hain Safflower Mayonnaise, or more, to your liking.
Whole organic Napa Cabbage
   or Lettuce leaves of choice

1. Place Eggs in cool, purified Water with a dash of salt. Bring Eggs to a boil, cover and let sit until cool enough to handle; this way they will be fully cooked, but not overcooked. Then peel.
2. Cut Eggs enough to be able to mash in bowl. Add Celery, Salt and Mayo.
3. Blend all Ingredients and spoon onto whole Napa Cabbage leaves, using them like a boat. If you want a wrap, use whole Lettuce leaves.
4. Sprinkle generously with Sunflower Seeds.

Success Secret: Toss a dash of salt into your Water while boiling eggs; it makes them easier to peel.

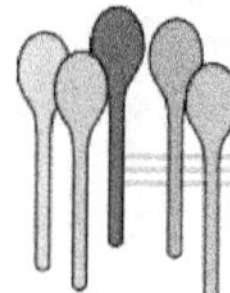

Variations

- If you don't eat Pickles due to the Vinegar and can't find naturally cured, try something like Olives or Capers and add Dill Weed for a Pickle-like flavor.
- Melt organic or European Brie on the Burger and keep warm while you sauté the organic Red Onion in the Oil left from the Burger, or use high-heat Oil or Bacon Grease.
- Toss organic Bleu Cheese and toasted organic Walnuts onto Salad before adding cooked Burger.

HAMBURGER SALAD

Love hamburgers but not the bun? Try this one for even more flavor. The bread won't absorb it all since there is none!

Serves: This recipe is measured in "per person" amounts.

Ingredients per person:
¼ lb or more ground protein
    (Hamburger, Ground Turkey or Veggie-burger)
Organic Salad greens
½ organic ripe Tomato
2 tsp organic White Onion
Anything else you love on Hamburgers,
    including Cheese, Bacon, etc.
Special Sauce (p. 46 or 63)

1. Grill Burger in patty or in pieces (I prefer the pieces, less work to do in cooking and eating. After flipping your cooked Burger, consider some soft Cheese if you like Cheeseburgers.
2. While Burger is cooking, arrange Salad Greens and other items on plate and coat with "Special Sauce" below. Then add whatever you like on your Hamburger from Pickles and Onions to Bacon and Mushrooms.

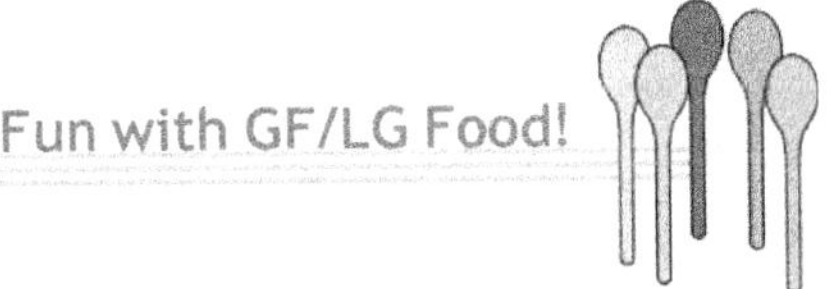

Vegans: Replace Safflower Mayonnaise with Vegan Mayo (p. 38).

SPECIAL SAUCE

The "Special Sauce" they use in most fast food restaurants is so simple it's unbelievable. This is how I think it's done and how it tastes right to me. Here you go:

Makes: About $^2/_3$ cup

Ingredients (Adjust to your personal taste):
    ¼ cup organic Ketchup or
        1 Tbsp. Tomato Paste, to avoid any sweeteners
    ½ cup Hain Safflower Mayonnaise
    1 tsp Celtic Sea Salt
        or 1 tsp Pink Himalayan Salt

1. Stir together all Ingredients and taste. Add whatever you like to make it taste the way you want it to.

Variation

- Use grilled, wild-caught Salmon instead of Chicken or pan-fry, browning first, then cooking at slow heat.

Vegans: Replace Chicken with vegan Protein of choice or sprouted/germinated Almonds, Seeds and Nuts.

Golden Chalice GINGER-SESAME SALAD with Marinated CHICKEN

Satisfying and savory, this favorite salad from our restaurant balances sweet, sour, spicy and crunchy in a delightful medley to please your senses, both visually and taste-wise. This is a wonderful, simple meal to honor any lunch guest in your home. I serve an appetizer of home-roasted, tamari-flavor almonds and cashews (p. 12). Everyone seems quite satisfied and no one wants bread, even when I offer it! I don't serve it as a matter of principle—but I do offer bread to my guests, and they seem to enjoy eating my healthy cuisine in its purity. They also know they need to save room for a smashing dessert! Any dessert from chapter five goes well with this meal.

Serves: This recipe is measured in "per person" amounts.

Ingredients per person:
    Organic Salad Greens to cover each guest's plate 3-
    4 oz. organic grilled
        or sautéed Chicken Breast
    1 Tbsp. toasted Organic Sesame Seeds (p. 12)
    ¼ cup organic Carrots, sliced thinly at angle, Asian style
    ¼ cup thinly sliced organic Red Bell Pepper
        (optional for nightshade-sensitive people)
    ¼ cup organic Bok Choy
        (optional—can also use Bean Sprouts, Chinese Pea Pods
        or Napa Cabbage) sliced thinly at angle, Asian style
    Ginger-Sesame Marinade
    Ginger-Sesame Salad Dressing (p. 30)

1. Two to three days before serving, and up to one week, marinate stir-fry sliced Chicken Breast (organic or natural —no hormones or antibiotics or free-range). Also, Amish or Hutterite Chicken is usually quite safe.

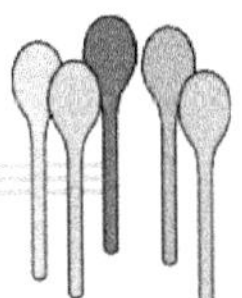

2. Just before serving, arrange Salad Greens on plate.
3. Slice as directed in Ingredients above and stir-fry quickly, just to heat, Red Bell Pepper, Bok Choy and Carrots. Keep just warm.
4. Stir fry Meat and place on top of each Salad. Arrange stir-fried Veggies around edges of Salad for decoration.
5. Sprinkle on Sesame Seeds, or place in bowl for your guests to do for themselves.
6. Serve immediately.

Ginger-Sesame Marinade

Serves: This recipe is measured in "per person" amounts.

Ingredients per person:
2 inches (or more, to your liking) organic Ginger Root, cut into chunks
2 Tbsp. organic Lemon Juice
  or, if you prefer, 2 Tbsp. organic Apple Cider
  or 2 Tbsp. Balsamic Vinegar
1 tsp organic toasted Sesame Oil
2 Tbsp. Braggs Liquid Amino Acids
$1/_8$ tsp Sweet Leaf Stevia
  or other form of Stevia, to taste
1 Tbsp. Unsweetened Apple Sauce

1. Blend all Ingredients until smooth. You're done!
2. Keep refrigerated, or use right away by covering cut up Meat or Fish. Marinate Chicken for up to one week. I like it marinated even longer, but you may not want flavor that intense.

Variations

- Top with toasted or sprouted Pine Nuts (Soak for at least four hours, then rinse) and grated Pecorino Romano Cheese (from Sheep) or organic Goat Feta Cheese, if you desire, just before serving.
- If you like Meat or Seafood, you may want to add sliced organic grilled or sautéed Chicken or Shrimp. Have Cayenne or Crushed Red Peppers available as condiments for friends who love it hot!
- If you are in a hurry or do not like Squash, feel free to use exclusively julienne Vegetables such as Zucchini, Red and Yellow Bell Peppers, Onions, etc. for a base instead of Spaghetti.

Vegans: Replace Ghee with pure virgin Coconut Oil. Add sprouted Nuts and Seeds or other Protein of choice.

Golden Chalice PESTO "UN-PASTA"

I used to love pasta, but since eating "un-pasta" for so long, it doesn't even appeal to me anymore! Now I love vegetables in their most flavorful outfits. Our guests at **The Golden Chalice** loved this dish, too.

Serves: Three to four people.

Ingredients:

- 1 medium organic Spaghetti Squash
- ½ cup thinly sliced organic Red Onion
- ½ cup julienne (cut lengthwise in thin strips) organic Red Bell Pepper
- 2 Tbsp. organic Ghee or 2 Tbsp. virgin Coconut Oil
- 1 cup organic Zucchini slices, julienne
- 3 Tbsp. organic Classic Pesto (p. 67 or 45)

1. Cut Spaghetti Squash in half and clean out seeds. (If you don't have a sharp enough knife to do this, simply bake whole and clean out seeds after baking.
2. Drizzle 1 Tbsp. of Ghee on each half, cover and bake at 350 °F for 30 minutes or more, depending on whether or not you like your un-pasta "al dente"—a little chewy. Scoop out 2 cups of Squash, which should now look somewhat like spaghetti. It's easier to keep in strands if you use a fork to take out.
3. Sauté Onion and Pepper in Oil of Choice or Ghee.
4. Add Zucchini to above and continue to sauté.
5. Add Spaghetti Squash and Pesto and blend in well.

Success Secret: Please adjust all amounts and measurements in this or any recipe to your personal taste.

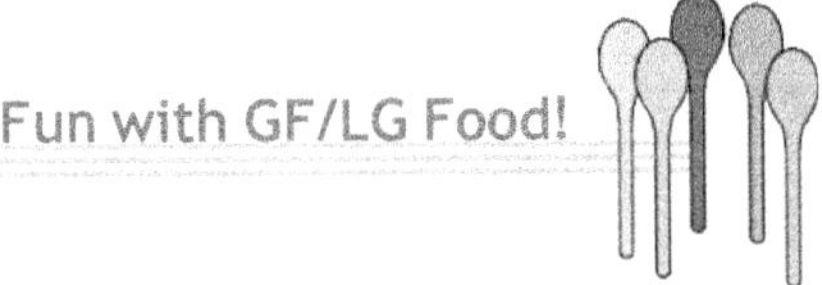

Variations

- Use organic roasted Walnuts instead of Pine Nuts.
- Use organic roasted or soaked Almonds instead of Pine Nuts.
- Use organic roasted Hazelnuts instead of Pine Nuts.
- I love this. I used Hazelnuts, Almonds and Walnuts all together because I was out of Pine Nuts and had very little of each. I was amazed at the yumminess.

Vegans and dairy-sensitive people: Replace Parmesan Cheese with vegan Cheese or simply add ½ tsp Celtic Sea or ½ tsp Pink Himalayan Salt.

CLASSIC PESTO

Makes: About 1 cup

Ingredients:
1 cup loosely packed fresh, washed organic Basil Leaves
¼ cup Pine Nuts
¼ cup shredded organic Parmesan Cheese
¼ cup organic cold-pressed, virgin Olive Oil

1. Blend in blender.

Success Secret: Fresh herbs create flavors that have more depth and can turn the simplest dish into a gourmet delight.

Variations

- Change the Vegetables to 1 cup organic Broccoli Stems in place of Bok Choy and Zucchini.
- Add unsweetened organic Coconut Milk or Water for thinner Sauce if it gets too thick. Stir to warm and serve with Quinoa or your own Grain choice or extra Veggies for low-glycemic meal. (Shredded or chopped organic Napa Cabbage is nice for base in place of Grains).
- For main dish: Add grilled Shrimp (sauté in pan until edges curl, then turn and do the same), grilled Chicken or other Meat marinated, if desired, using Lemon based Marinade, p. 39 or 49) stir-fried in virgin, hand-pressed Coconut Oil.

Vegans: For extra protein, top with ½ cup organic roasted or soaked, germinated Cashews, Sunflower and/or Pumpkin Seeds.

Nut-sensitive people: Try replacing Cashews with organic Sunflower Seeds.

Golden Chalice
LEMON CASHEW CURRY

A warm dish for rainy days, the Lemon Cashew Curry can be made as hot as you want with your favorite curry paste. The recipe below is mildly flavored for a more delicate palate, allowing you to enjoy the flavors of the lemon and vegetables.

Serves: One to two people

Ingredients:
   ½ cup soaked organic Cashews
       (soak for four hours or more, then rinse)
   ½ cup pure Water
   ¼ tsp organic Curry Powder
   ¼ tsp organic Cumin Powder
   2 tsp Braggs Liquid Amino Acids
   ¼ tsp Celtic Sea Salt
       or ¼ tsp Pink Himalayan Salt
   2 Tbsp. organic Lemon Juice
   ½ Tbsp. organic Lemon Zest
   ½ cup angle-sliced organic Carrots
   ¼ cup chopped organic Onion
   ½ cup angle-sliced organic Bok Choy
   ½ cup angle-sliced organic Zucchini
   Tamari-flavor Roasted Cashews (p. 12)

1. Blend in blender (for Sauce); Cashews, Water, Curry, Cumin, Braggs Aminos, Salt, Lemon Juice and Zest.
2. Chop and stir fry in wok or pan: Carrots, Onion, Bok Choy, Zucchini.
3. Add Sauce to Veggie mixture.
4. Garnish with Tamari-flavor Roasted Cashews.

Success Secret: A balance of sweet flavors (can be carrots or other vegetables like red peppers) and salty, as well as soft and crunchy textures make delicious meals.

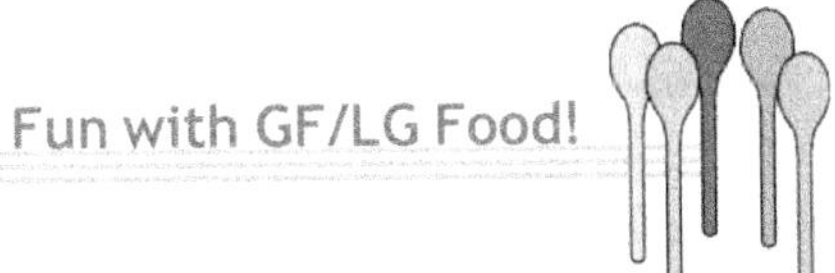

Variations

- For creamier sauce, add 1 Tbsp. Hain Safflower Mayonnaise.
- Add 1 Tbsp. organic Pesto for a more exotic flavor.
- Add ½ cup julienne organic Red Bell Pepper.
- Try using Spaghetti Squash (see p. 66 for instructions on baking)

Vegans: Replace Seafood with organic Sprouted Nuts and/or Seeds (p. 13) or another vegan Protein. Use Vegan Mayo (p. 38).

Un-PASTA de ATLANTIS (Seafood Un-pasta)

Seafood pasta has always been a favorite of mine and so simple to make. People rave about it, and it only takes a few short minutes to make! But I don't eat pasta anymore due to the high glycemic level, even when it is gluten-free. So those of you who are of like mind (or should I say "like stomach"?) may enjoy the healthy alternative below. For a romantic dinner that is stress-free and impresses greatly, try this recipe with a simple, colorful salad (I'd suggest the Kalamata Olive Salad Dressing p. 33) and a premade dessert (chapter 5).

Serves: Two to three people

Ingredients:
- 1 clove crushed fresh organic Garlic
- 2 Tbsp. organic Ghee
  - or 2 Tbsp. Butter
  - or 2 Tbsp. Butter-flavored alternative
- 1 Tbsp. organic Lemon Juice
- 1 tsp fresh organic Lemon Zest
- 1 tsp dried organic Parsley
  - or 1 tablespoon fresh organic Parsley
- ¼ tsp Celtic Sea Salt, to taste
  - or ¼ tsp Pink Himalayan Salt, to taste
- 2 cups organic Zucchini, julienne (sliced lengthwise in very thin strips or in food processor)—this is in place of traditional Pasta
- ½ to 1 cup raw or precooked wild-caught Seafood such as: Crab, Shrimp and/or Scallops (look for the kind without chemical additives).

1. Blend together and warm: Garlic, Ghee, Lemon Juice, Lemon Zest, Parsley and Salt until Ghee or Butter is melted and garlic slightly cooked.
2. Add Zucchini and Seafood (unless precooked) to garlic mixture and slightly sauté.
3. Add pre-cooked Seafood to Garlic mixture. Toss.

Vegans: Replace Chicken with organic Sprouted Nuts and/or Seeds (p. 13) or other vegan Protein.

Golden Chalice
ITALIAN CHICKEN SALAD

Serves: Eight to 10 people

Ingredients:

    1 lb. organic Chicken, cooked
       (use leftover Chicken—see p. 20)
    1 cup organic chopped Tomatoes
    ¼ cup sliced, pitted organic Kalamata Olives
    2 Tbsp. organic Pesto
    1 cup Hain Safflower Mayonnaise
    1 cup organic Artichoke Hearts
      (non-marinated bottled have better flavor)
    ½ cup organic Bok Choy

1. Chop Chicken and Tomatoes in small squares. Cut Artichoke Hearts in small wedges.
2. Blend all Ingredients in large bowl and serve or refrigerate.

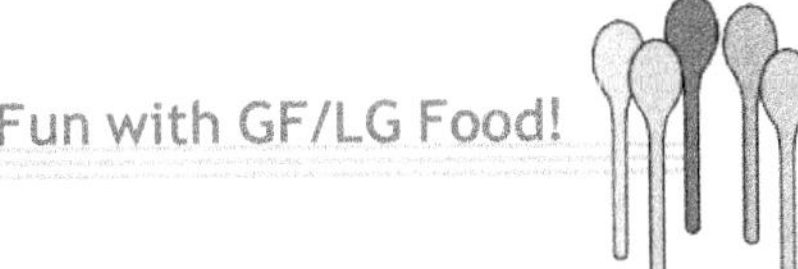

Variations

- Top with toasted organic Sesame Seeds. Toast Seeds in pan or in oven 350 °F for about 5 minutes or less. Watch carefully and stir every few minutes.
- Use *Golden Chalice* House Dressing (p. 34) as marinade instead of the Ginger Dressing. Leave out the Oil and replace the oregano with organic Lemon Zest. Reserve 1 Tbsp. to add to Vegetables just before removing from heat.
- Blend ¼ cup Braggs Liquid Amino Acids with ¼ cup Unsweetened Apple Sauce and ¼ tsp Sweet Leaf Stevia. Use as Marinade instead of the Ginger Dressing. Reserve 1 Tbsp. to add to Vegetables just before removing from heat.
- Add any of the variations to a salad. You can also use the Sweet Wasabi Dressing (p. 37).

Vegans: Replace animal protein with organic Sprouted Nuts and/or Seeds (p. 13) or other vegan Protein.

Golden Chalice
STIR FRY

Serves: This recipe is measured in "per person" amounts.

Ingredients per person (or use proportions to your liking):

    1 Tbsp. organic, virgin cold-pressed Coconut Oil
       or 1 Tbsp. other high-heat Oil
    ½ oz Onion
    1 oz Carrots
    1 oz Snow peas
    1 oz Zucchini
    2 oz Bok Choy
    2 oz Chinese Cabbage
    3-4 oz Shrimp
       or 3-4 oz Chicken
       or 3-4 oz Beef
       or 3-4 oz Sprouted Almonds, marinated 24 hours minimum in Ginger-Sesame Marinade (p. 65). Use enough to cover Meat or Fish or Nuts
    1 Tbsp. Fresh Ginger-Sesame Dressing (p. 30)

1. Cut all Vegetables at an angle, like you see in Asian restaurants.
2. Begin with the Vegetables at the top of the list (less likely to overcook) and toss into Oil at high heat, stirring quickly.
3. Toss with Ginger Dressing, remove vegetables and keep warm. Stir-fry marinated seafood or meat of choice (do not cook Almonds) and place over vegetables.

Variations

- Add grilled or roasted organic Red Bell Pepper strips.
- For color without nightshades, add thin julienne organic Red Beets and/or Carrots.
- Use or offer Sweet Wasabi Salad Dressing (p. 37) for those who like it hot!

Golden Chalice
AHI TUNA SALAD

Do you love fresh fish? I do, but only if it's salmon, halibut, ahi tuna or other Hawaiian fish. My tastes are expensive! This recipe can be adapted to any of these.

Serves: This recipe is measured in "per person" amounts.

Ingredients per person:
3-4 oz. wild-caught Ahi Tuna
1 Tbsp. organic virgin cold-pressed Coconut Oil
   or 1 Tbsp. other high-heat Oil
Ginger-Sesame Marinade (p. 65)
   —Enough to cover fish
Ginger-Sesame Dressing
Fresh organic Spring Greens
Toasted organic Sesame Seeds (see variations, p. 12)

1. 24 hours ahead of serving, cut Ahi Tuna in strips, then cover with Marinade.
2. Arrange Salad Greens on plate and place toasted Sesame Seeds in small serving bowl with small spoon for guests to sprinkle over Salad to their liking.
3. Sear Ahi Tuna in Oil at medium temperature. Turn stove off just when turning fish, so that it does not get overdone. Let it cook through unless you have Sushi-grade Fish.
4. Arrange Tuna on top of salad and serve with Fresh Ginger-Sesame Salad Dressing (p. 30).

Success Secret: You may think that fish are salty enough by themselves, but trust me, unless they are pickled or smoked (lots of salt already added) they taste way better with salt added! Simple, humble salt is the secret of many fine chefs. They often use kosher or some other high quality salt. Celtic sea salt and Pink Himalayan salt are the very healthiest and the tastiest!

Variations

- Use organic Almonds instead of Sesame Seeds. Grind in Blender or nut-grinder.
- Use organic Cashews instead of Sesame Seeds. Grind in blender or nut-grinder.
- Use Pine Nuts and Pesto instead of Sesame Seeds.
- Use Seeds or Nuts of your choice adding 1 tsp crushed dry organic Herbs. If you like Italian flavors, use Italian Herbs like Oregano, Thyme, Rosemary and Basil.
- For more subtle flavors, use Tarragon (good with Fish) or Rosemary.
- Use Seeds or Nuts of your choice, adding 1 tsp organic Lemon or Orange Zest. Try mixing the flavors with Herbs. Lemon-Tarragon is good.

SEED ENCRUSTED FISH OF YOUR CHOICE

Okay, I'll eat other white fish like walleye on occasion if I know it's from a fairly clean lake and I can dress it up. I used to love breaded fish, especially if it was crunchy, but nuts or seeds enhance the flavor for me and hopefully for you too. And they can be crunchy, too!

Serves: One to four people (depending on appetites)

Ingredients:

½ lb fresh, cleaned Walleye or other favorite Fish
½ cup organic unhulled Sesame Seeds
½ tsp Celtic Sea Salt
    or ½ tsp Pink Himalayan Salt
1 organic Egg

1. Beal Egg.
2. Grind or crush Sesame Seeds (can use dedicated coffee grinder).
3. Drag Fish through Egg on both sides, using clean rubber gloves or clean hands to get a good grip and so as not to tear Fish (utensils would).
4. Sprinkle crushed Seeds on Fish, turn and cover other side as well. Don't worry if some fall off, etc. They make yummy tidbits!
5. Coat bottom of pan with Oil or Ghee.
6. Bake uncovered at 300 °F. Check it at 15 minutes, then check every 5 minutes to see if done. You can tell by putting a fork into the Fish and pulling gently. If it flakes, it's done. Be careful not to overcook.

Success Secret: Cooking time depends on thickness of cut. If part of the cut is thinner than another, check it first, then cut it off and keep it warm, if necessary so it doesn't get overcooked with the rest of the fish.

Variations

- Replace or add Broccoli to Mushrooms. Peel and chop Broccoli stems. Don't use tops, unless you pre-cook them.
- Replace Mushrooms with small strips of organic Roasted Red Bell Pepper (p. 7).
- Replace Mushrooms with equal parts sliced organic Olives and chopped organic fresh or sun-dried Tomato (soaked overnight).
- Add organic Pesto, Olive Oil or Marinara Sauce. to the Olive and Tomato Frittata above.
- Top with Cheese of choice.
- Your turn! Use your imagination. If you've been reading these recipes, you may be coming up with ideas that fit your health scheme. Go for it! The only way is to try things until you strike gold!

SHITAKE MUSHROOM FRITTATA

Frittatas are Italian omelets, but for some reason (a European name, maybe?), they are approved as dinner food! Or lunch.

Serves: This recipe is measured in "per person" amounts.

Ingredients per person:

½ cup organic Shitake Mushrooms
1 Tbsp. organic White Onion
1 extra large organic Egg
Dash Celtic Sea Salt
    or dash Pink Himalayan Salt
Dash Pepper (optional)
1 tsp Ghee
    or 1 tsp Oil of Choice
$\frac{1}{8}$ tsp Parsley

1. Finely chop Onions and coarsely slice Mushrooms. Then sauté Mushrooms and Onions in Ghee or Oil.
2. While Veggies are cooking, scramble Egg and Salt/Pepper or whip in blender for fluffier Frittata.
3. When Mushrooms and Onions are cooked, add Egg to pan and mix in with Veggies. Let cook like Omelet, cooking through, or bake in oven at 350 °F until done. Check after five minutes and look for light browning on edges.
4. Serve immediately or keep warm at very low heat for just a few minutes at most.

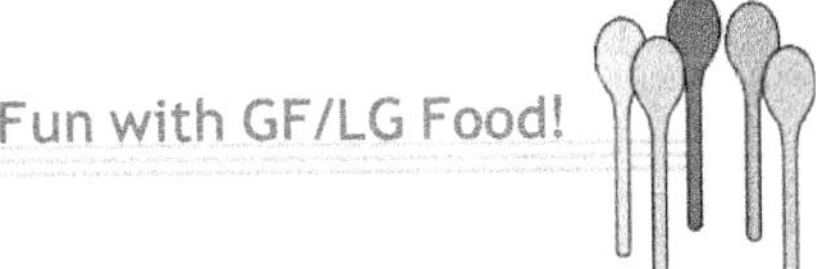

Variations

- Add ½ cup sautéed organic Shitake Mushrooms
- Add ½ cup organic sautéed chopped Onions
- Add 1 clove crushed organic sautéed Garlic
- Add 1 tsp organic Sage and Thyme to make it taste like stuffing!

Vegans: Replace Drippings or Broth with Braggs Liquid Amino Acids.

Bonus for Gravy-Lovin' Lords and Ladies

QUICK GRAVY

Serves: This recipe is measured in "per cup" amounts.

Ingredients per cup:

1 cup Meat Drippings
   or 1 cup Broth
   or 1 cup Braggs Liquid Amino Acids—if no broth is available
1 tsp Arrowroot Powder
½ tsp Celtic Sea Salt
   or ½ tsp Pink Himalayan Salt
Organic White, to taste
   or Black Pepper, to taste

1. Stir salt into liquid, then Arrowroot Powder into cool or just warm liquid (not hot).
2. Bring to a simmer, stirring constantly. Remove from heat as soon as it is thick enough for you. If you want it thicker, mix more Arrowroot Powder with just enough pure Water to make it melt, then mix with liquid on stove and heat once more until thick enough.
3. Add Pepper last.

Success Secret: Pepper is best for digestive system when not cooked because then it can be an irritant.

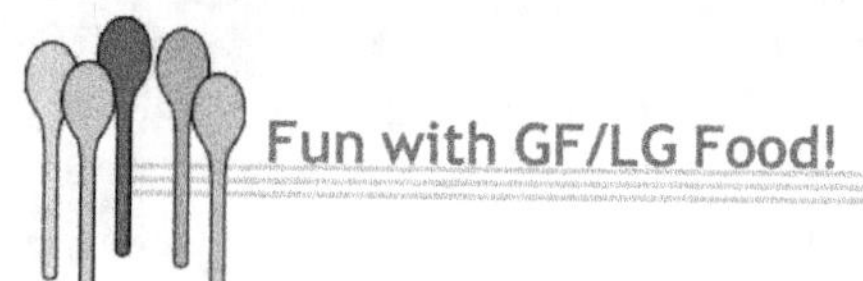

Notes

Chapter 5
Delectable Desserts

These desserts are not very sweet, so if you like yours more sweet, you may add more stevia leaf extract or raw, powdered stevia leaf (available in health food stores).

Recipes beginning with the words *"Golden Chalice"* are from my former gluten-free, diabetic-friendly restaurant of the same name.

Golden Chalice
CARROT CAKE

I've been asked for this recipe more times than I can remember, as everyone loves it. The key is the moisture, which is obtained by the high oil content—and it's healthy oil, so stay calm! This cake is very moist and tastes delicious by itself, but try the Cream Cheese Frosting recipe or Sweet Cashew Cream (p. 41 or 80) if you are vegan or have dairy sensitivities. Personally, I like it just as well unfrosted...you get all the spiciness, yum! Or, use Coconut Milk (thick part).
Makes: About 2 cups

> **Success Secret:**
> Desserts are more flavorful when not too sweet. Using either Unsweetened Apple Sauce as a sweetener is lower-glycemic.

Vegans: Replace Egg with Egg Substitute or try 1 tsp Arrowroot Powder to hold cake or brownies together.

Nut-sensitive people: Replace Almond Meal Flour with any gluten-free Flour then cover 5 minutes after baking so it stays moist.

In place of Sweet Cashew Cream in any recipe, try Coconut Milk, found in health food and Asian stores. Use the creamy part which has risen to the top of the can. You can flavor and sweeten it to taste the same way you would Sweet Cashew Cream.

Wheat and gluten-sensitive people: Read all labels when buying grains to be sure they don't say "May contain wheat."

Coconut Flour is a good alternative to other Flours you may not be able to use.

Makes: One 9" x 9" cake

Ingredients:
- 1½ cup Almond Meal Flour
- ½ cup organic Quinoa or Amaranth Flour
    or combination of these
- 2 tsp aluminum-free Baking Powder (health food store)
- 2 tsp organic Cinnamon
- Organic Spices: ¼ tsp each organic Allspice and Cloves
- 1 tsp Celtic Sea Salt
    or 1 tsp Pink Himalayan Salt
- 1 cup virgin Coconut Oil or Ghee,
    or ½ and ½ of each
- ½ tsp Sweet Leaf Stevia, to taste
    or other form of Stevia, to taste
- 1 cup Unsweetened Apple Sauce
- 1 tsp organic Vanilla Extract
    or 1 tsp Vanilla Flavor (Celiacs may not tolerate extract)
- 3 cups grated Carrots
    (try to get sweet carrots if not adding sweetener)
- 4 Eggs
- ½ cup chopped organic Walnuts (optional)

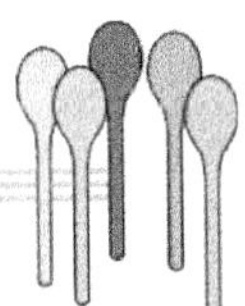

1. Preheat oven to 350 °F. Grease and flour 9" x 9" x 2" pan.
2. Mix together: Almond Meal or Flours, Baking Powder, Cinnamon, Allspice, Cloves and Salt.
3. Blend in Oil or Ghee, Stevia, Unsweetened Apple Sauce and Vanilla.
4. Add grated Carrots, then Eggs, one at a time, beating well after each addition.
5. Optional: Blend in Walnuts
6. Bake 30-40 minutes or till done. Cool and cover after 5 to 10 minutes to maintain moisture if using Flours other than Nut Meal. You can frost with Cream Cheese frosting or Sweet Cashew Cream.
7. Serve warm if not frosted or at room temperature with Cream Cheese Frosting. Refrigerate if not serving until next day or if leftovers, but return to room temperature to serve.

CREAM CHEESE FROSTING

Makes: Enough frosting for a 9" x 9" cake

Ingredients:
    8 oz softened organic Cream Cheese
    I tsp organic Vanilla Extract
        or I tsp Vanilla Flavor (Celiacs may not tolerate extract)
    1 Tbsp. organic pure Maple Syrup
        or ¼ cup Unsweetened Apple Sauce
    ½ tsp Sweet Leaf Stevia, to taste
        or other form of Stevia, to taste

1. Mix together all ingredients until smooth. Spread immediately on cooled cake or refrigerate, then before frosting cake, let warm up to room temperature.
2. (Optional) Add a little purified Water to stretch the amount and to make frosting softer and easier to blend and frost cake.

Nut-sensitive people: In place of organic cream or Sweet Cashew Cream in any recipe, try Coconut Milk, found in health food and Asian stores. Use the creamy part which has risen to the top of the can. You can flavor and sweeten it to taste the same way you would Sweet Cashew Cream.

Golden Chalice
SWEET CASHEW CREAM (Vegan)

For those who like a smooth, creamy alternative to dairy creams.

Makes: About ¾ cup

Ingredients:
   ½ cup organic Cashews, germinated
      (soaked for eight hours and rinsed well—becomes $^2/_3$ cup
      after soaking—use within two days, rinse daily)
   ¼ cup purified Water
   2 dashes Celtic Sea Salt
      or 2 dashes Pink Himalayan Salt
   1 tsp organic Vanilla Extract
      or 1 tsp Vanilla Flavor (Celiacs may not tolerate extract)
   1 Tbsp. organic pure Maple Syrup
      or ¼ cup Unsweetened Apple Sauce
   ½ tsp Sweet Leaf Stevia, to taste
      or other form of Stevia, to taste

1. Blend all ingredients in blender or food processor until smooth.
2. Refrigerate or use immediately. Freeze unused portion within 2 days.

Success Secret: When you combine fruit and stevia in recipes for sweetening, the result tastes more like sugar. I've never had anyone notice the stevia flavor by doing that.

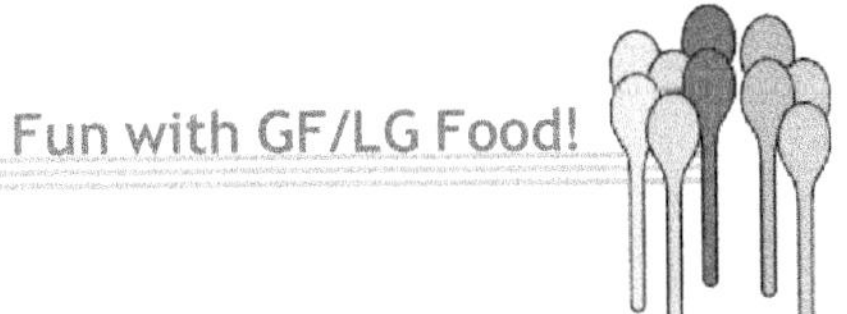

Vegans: Replace Egg with Egg Substitute.

Dairy-sensitive people: Replace Butter or Ghee with organic, virgin Coconut Oil .

Nut-sensitive people: Replace Almond Meal Flour with any gluten-free Flour.

Success Secret: Keep spices in freezer to maintain full flavor, freshness. Use organic if possible, buy small amounts to maintain freshness.

CHUNKY APPLE CAKE

This is a fun combination of cake and pie.

Makes: One 9" x 9" cake

Ingredients:

    1½ cups Almond Meal Flour
    2 Tbsps. Protein Powder of Choice (holds
       together better)
    ½ cup organic Quinoa or Amaranth Flour
       or combination of these
    2 tsp aluminum-free Baking Soda (health food store)
    1 tsp organic Cinnamon
    ½ tsp each Organic Spices:
       Allspice and Nutmeg,
    ¼ tsp Organic Cloves
    ¼ tsp Celtic Sea Salt
       or ¼ tsp Pink Himalayan Salt
    ½ cup (one stick) softened, melted organic Butter
       or ½ cup organic Ghee (clarified butter)
    ½ tsp organic Stevia leaf, to taste
       or Sweet Leaf Stevia extract, to taste
    ½ cup organic Unsweetened Apple Sauce
    I tsp organic Vanilla Extract
       or I tsp Vanilla Flavor (Celiacs may not tolerate extract)
    2 organic Eggs
    2 cups chopped organic Apples,
       cut in approximately ½ inch cubes
    1 cup organic Walnuts (optional)
Cream Cheese Frosting (optional, p. 79)

1. Preheat oven to 350 °F. Grease and flour 9" x 9" x 2" pan.
2. Mix together Flours, Baking Soda, Spices and Salt.
3. Blend in Ghee or Oil, Stevia, Unsweetened Apple Sauce
   , Vanilla and Eggs. Mix well, 200 strokes with fork or 2
   minutes with electric mixer.
4. Gently blend in Apples and Walnuts. (Nuts are optional.)
5. Bake 50 minutes or until done. Cool and serve plain or
   with Cream Cheese Frosting.

Vegans: Replace Eggs with a combination of Protein Powder, soaked Cashews or Almond Meal, plus a small amount of Water and Egg Substitute of your choice.

Or instead of Egg Substitute, add 1 tsp or more Arrowroot Powder, according to how firm you like your pancakes. Replace Ghee with virgin Coconut Oil or Oil of Choice to fry pancakes.
Making these pancakes very small works best.

Dairy-sensitive people:
Replace Cottage Cheese with 1 cup soaked Cashews (see Sweet Cashew Cream recipe, p. 41 or 80) for instructions on soaking/germinating). Replace Butter with ½ cup Coconut Oil.

Nut-sensitive people: In place of organic cream or Sweet Cashew Cream in any recipe, try Coconut Milk, found in health food and Asian stores. Use the creamy part which has risen to the top of the can. You can flavor and sweeten it to taste the same way you would Sweet Cashew Cream.

LOW-CARB DESSERT CRÊPES

This recipe is also in the main dishes chapter—same one, so you can think of it for a main course as well as a dessert. I learned from a French Canadian friend how to make these. You really can't go wrong if you have a well-greased or naturally non-stick pan. The consistency is very thin, but you can make it thicker (for heavier crêpes) by adding more flour.

Serves: Eight to ten people

Ingredients:
One cup organic Cottage Cheese, Ricotta Cheese (or cheese substitute)
6 organic or free-range Eggs
½ cup Amaranth or Quinoa Flour
½ tsp Celtic Sea Salt
    or ½ tsp Pink Himalayan Salt
I tsp aluminum-free Baking Powder (health food store)
I tsp organic Vanilla Extract
    or I tsp Vanilla Flavor (Celiacs may not tolerate extract)
½ cup Ghee, Butter
    or ½ cup virgin Coconut Oil
    or ½ cup Oil of Choice
I Tbsp. Lemon Zest
(peel) 1 tsp organic
Cinnamon
¼ tsp organic Almond Extract
    or ¼ tsp Almond Flavor (Celiacs may not tolerate extract) Banana Orange Sauce or Fruit Sauce of choice

1. Blend all ingredients in blender.
2. Add ¼ cup purified Water or more to blender, depending on the thickness you'd like for the Crêpes. Test a small one first. Make sure your pan is well greased unless it is non-stick (not recommended unless titanium, for health reasons—see p. 120). Spread on pan with a large spoon, unless you are an expert crêpe- maker.

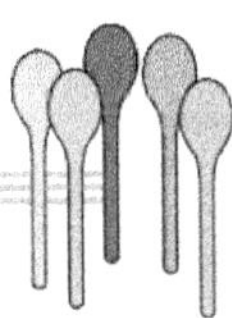

1. If batter is too thin, add soaked Cashews to firm up, or add more Flour, 1 Tbsp. at a time.
2. Top with Banana-Orange Sauce or Fruit Sauce of choice.

BLUEBERRY-LEMON SAUCE

Variations

- Instead of Lemon Zest or Extract, mix in organic Strawberries or Cherries. Any of the Fruit can be frozen as well as fresh.
- Instead of Lemon Zest or Extract, add organic tropical Fruit of your choice and organic, unsweetened, shredded Coconut.
- Replace both Blueberries and Lemon Zest or Flavor with 1½ to 2 cups of other Fruit of your choice.
- Use organic fresh Apples of your choice. Sweet Apples require less added sweetener.

Very versatile, you can make this into any kind of Fruit Sauce you wish.

Serves: About 2 cups

Ingredients:

¼ cup organic Ghee (clarified Butter)
½ to 2 cups Blueberries
½ cup organic Unsweetened Apple Sauce
1 cup or more Purified Water
1 tsp organic Vanilla Extract
   or I tsp Vanilla Flavor (Celiacs may not tolerate extract)
½ tsp organic Lemon Extract
   or Grated Peel of ½ organic Lemon
½ tsp Celtic Sea Salt
   or ½ tsp Pink Himalayan Salt
¼ tsp Stevia of choice and either
   Unsweetened Apple Sauce,
   or organic Maple Syrup, to taste

1. Melt Ghee in medium-size Saucepan:
2. Add blueberries and Raisins to hot Ghee, sauté for about one minute.
3. Add Water, Extracts, Salt, Stevia and Unsweetened Apple Sauce or Maple Syrup if you like.
4. Do taste and use your own sweetness meter!
5. Simmer for 5 minutes, then serve hot. Refrigerate leftovers. (Ha! Doubt there will be any.)

Important Note: This sauce is fairly thin, as I like my sauce to seep into my pancakes. To thicken your sauce simply blend 1 Tbsp. Arrowroot into the Water first, then stir constantly until thickened.

Vegans: Replace Ghee with cold-pressed virgin Coconut Oil.

Nut-sensitive people: Replace Almond Meal Flour with 1 cup Amaranth Flour and add extra oil—¼ cup or more as needed to stick together.

Golden Chalice CHERRY-ALMOND TART

If you love Cherries, you'll love this dessert, as did all of our guests at ***The Golden Chalice Restaurant and Gallery.***

Makes: One 9" pie

Ingredients:

Gluten-Free Crust

  2 Tbsp. Ghee
  ¼ tsp Celtic Sea Salt
    or ¼ tsp Pink Himalayan Salt
  ¼ cup Amaranth Flour
  ¾ cup Almond Meal/Flour, finely ground
    —buy or grind your own in blender
  1 Egg or Egg Replacer (add 1 Tbsp. Protein Powder if using Egg Replacer

1. Melt Ghee or Coconut Oil on low heat (right in 9" pie pan, if you want to wash fewer pans).
2. Mix in Almond Meal, Amaranth or Coconut Flour, Salt and Egg or Egg Replacer with Protein Powder, if you use it, right in pie pan.

    Important Note: mix until mixture clumps together, so the Oil spreads evenly and will press well into pan and stay more firm.

3. Press into pie pan.

Filling:

20 oz frozen organic Sweet Black Cherries
¼ to ½ cup Unsweetened Apple Sauce
    or ¼ to ½ cup unsweetened organic Cherry
    or ¼ to ½ cup unsweetened organic Apple Juice
1 Tbsp. Agar-Agar (the no starch choice)
    or 1 Tbsp. Arrowroot Powder
I tsp organic Vanilla Extract
½ tsp Almond Extract
⅛ tsp Celtic Sea Salt
    or ⅛ tsp Pink Himlayan Salt
⅛ tsp Stevia of choice
½ tsp Ghee or Coconut Oil
½ cup slivered or ground Almonds

1. Thaw and drain liquid from Cherries. Drain well, into easy-pour container; then gently press Cherries in sieve to release most of the Juice without crushing the Cherries too much. Pour liquid into 1 cup measuring container.
2. Add Unsweetened Apple Sauce , Cherry or Apple Juice to the Juice from frozen, drained Cherries to make up 1 cup total liquid.
3. Pour liquid into saucepan, then add Agar-Agar, Arrowroot Powder and follow directions for whichever thickener you use. (Heat and stir until bubbling and thickened, stirring constantly. If using Agar Agar, continue to boil for 4 minutes.)
4. Add Vanilla Extract, Almond Extract, Salt, Stevia and Ghee or Coconut Oil.
5. Blend above mixture with Cherries and pour into crust of your choice.
6. Top with slivered or ground organic Almonds and bake at 350 °F for 15 to 20 minutes or until Almonds are slightly browned. Cool and refrigerate to firm. Serve later at room temperature in winter, cooled in summer.

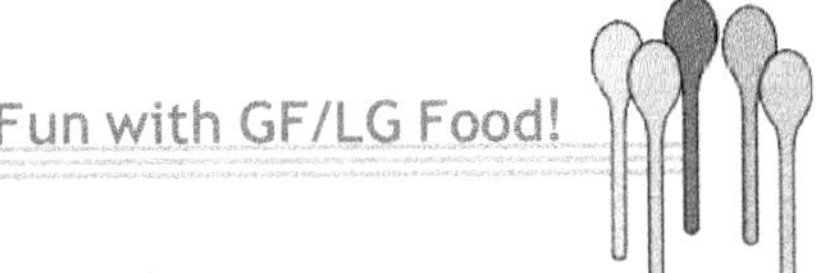

APPLE OR PEACH COBBLER

This old-fashioned recipe is quite tasty, yet simple to make.

Makes: One 9" x 9" cobbler

Ingredients:

Filling
1 Tbsp. organic Ghee
    or 1 Tbsp. organic Butter
    or 1 Tbsp. cold-pressed virgin Coconut
Oil 3 large or 5 small organic sweet Apples
    or 3 large or 5 small organic ripe Peaches
½ tsp Sweet Leaf Stevia, to taste
    or other form of Stevia, to taste
1 tsp organic Vanilla Extract
    or 1 tsp Vanilla Flavor (Celiacs may not tolerate extract)
¼ cup Unsweetened Apple Sauce

For Apple cobbler only, add:
1 tsp Lemon Juice
1 tsp organic Cinnamon
¼ tsp organic Allspice

1. Preheat oven to 350 °F.
2. Melt Ghee, Butter or Coconut Oil.
3. Wash and thinly slice Apples (no need to peel, as that is the best part for your health!) or Peaches.
4. Blend in remaining ingredients.
5. Place cobbler filling into 9" x 9" x 2" pan and spread with topping.
6. Bake for about 30 minutes or until topping is just brown.

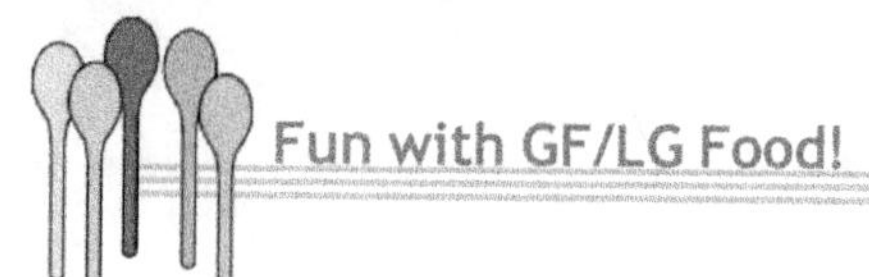

Topping

    ¼ cup melted Ghee
      or ¼ cup Oil
  1 cup ground organic Nuts or Seeds of any kind
      or 1 cup gluten-free Flour
  ¼ cup Amaranth or Quinoa Flour, if desired,
      for a more solid crust on top
  ½ tsp Sweet Leaf Stevia Extract, to taste
      or other form of Stevia, to taste

1. Mix together first three ingredients, then add Stevia and spread on cobbler filling before baking.

COCONUT MACAROONS

Makes: ½ to 1 dozen cookies, depending on size.

Ingredients:

$^1/_3$ cup organic Quinoa Flour

¼ tsp Baking Powder

$^2/_3$ cup dried, grated organic Coconut

2 Tbsp. melted, unsalted organic Butter

     or 2 Tbsp. melted Ghee

     or 2 Tbsp. melted Coconut Oil

1 Tbsp. organic Maple Syrup

½ tsp Sweet Leaf Stevia Extract, to taste

     or other form of Stevia, to taste

1 tsp organic Vanilla Extract

     or 1 tsp Vanilla Flavor (Celiacs may not tolerate extract)

¼ tsp organic Almond Extract

     or 1 tsp Almond Flavor (Celiacs may not tolerate extract)

2 organic Egg Whites

¼ tsp Celtic Sea Salt (to stiffen)

     or ¼ tsp Pink Himalayan Salt (to stiffen)

1. Preheat oven to 325 °F and mix together Flour, Baking Powder and Coconut.
2. Add melted Butter, Ghee or Coconut Oil and Sweeteners and Extracts.
3. Whip Egg Whites and Salt until stiff.
4. Fold Egg mixture into batter and drop onto greased cookie sheets, baking for 15-20 minutes.

Variations

- For a more classic Brownie taste, instead of Coconut, use toasted organic Walnuts, same amounts, and no almond butter.
- For an Orange-Chocolate flavor, add 1 tsp Orange Extract and/or 1 Tbsp. organic Orange Zest.
- If you can eat all Nuts and Seeds, you can make this with the Coconut, organic toasted Nuts and Seeds and Almond Butter, but no Carob Powder. Simply use recipe above, but replace Carob and Chicory with more ground Nuts of your choice.

People with extra sensitive diets: This recipe is very versatile for special diets, even without fruit, because Carob powder is naturally sweet. You can eliminate the Apple Sauce and simply use Stevia, Carob Powder and Seeds/Nuts of choice with Vanilla Extract or Flavor and a little Water or melted Coconut Oil. Most any diet can handle that.

Golden Chalice CAROB-COCONUT TRUFFLES

A mostly raw-food dessert, this is a favorite among my friends. Soak organic Almonds in purified Water overnight to bring out the full nutritional value in this dessert. Rinse well and grind in blender.

Serves: Three to five people

Ingredients:

1 tablespoon hand-pressed virgin Coconut Oil, melted
¼ cup organic Unsweetened Apple Sauce
    or simply use more Stevia
1 cup organic Unsweetened Coconut, dry, shredded
1 tablespoon organic Almond Butter
¼ tsp organic Almond Extract
    or ¼ tsp Almond Flavor (Celiacs may not tolerate extract)
I tsp organic Vanilla Extract
    or I tsp Vanilla Flavor (Celiacs may not tolerate extract)
⅛ tsp Celtic Sea Salt
    or ⅛ tsp Pink Himlayan Salt (if unsalted Almond Butter)
2 tablespoons organic Carob Powder—either raw or roasted
2 tablespoons organic Roasted Chicory root, finely ground
    (use blender or coffee grinder if necessary)—gives more
    of a chocolatey flavor
½ cup soaked, chopped organic Almonds
    —soak 16 hours, rinse every 8 hours

1. Even though Coconut is shredded, grind finely in dedicated coffee grinder (one not used for coffee).
2. Blend all ingredients except ¼ cup ground Coconut together in small bowl.
3. Roll into balls, sizing as you wish (we used golf-ball size at the restaurant) then roll in the ¼ cup ground organic Coconut. It looks and feels almost like Powdered Sugar, but it is much better for you!

Variations

- Use Blueberries instead of Strawberries.
- Use Cherries instead of Strawberries.
- Use Mango, Pineapple, Bananas, Coconut and Papaya or any combination thereof instead of Strawberries.
- Mix up any Fruit you want!
- Top with toasted organic Pecan or Almond Pieces.

Vegans: Replace Whipped Cream with Sweet Cashew Cream—but simply use less Water to make it thicker).

Nut-sensitive people: In place of organic cream or Sweet Cashew Cream in any recipe, try Coconut Milk, found in health food and Asian stores. Use the creamy part which has risen to the top of the can. You can flavor and sweeten it to taste the same way you would Sweet Cashew Cream.

STRAWBERRIES AND WHIPPED CREAM with COULIS

Great picnic dish, because it only needs to stay cool, not frozen as ice cream does.

Serves: Two to four people

Ingredients:

    2 quarts fresh, ripe organic Strawberries
    Whipped Cream
        or Sweet Cashew Cream (p. 41 or 80)
    Strawberry Coulis

1. Wash Strawberries and slice.
2. At picnic site or just before serving, portion out Strawberries and top with Whipped Cream or Cashew Cream, then the Coulis.

WHIPPED CREAM

Makes: 2-3 cups

Ingredients:

    1 pint organic Whipping Cream
    1 Tbsp. pure organic Maple Syrup
    ½ tsp Sweet Leaf Stevia Liquid, to taste
        or other form of Stevia, to taste
    I tsp organic Vanilla Extract
        or I tsp Vanilla Flavor (Celiacs may not tolerate extract)

1. Whip until firm.

STRAWBERRY COULIS

Serves: Two to four people

Ingredients:
  1 pint fresh organic Strawberries
     for topping over the Whipped Cream
  1 cup organic Unsweetened Apple
Sauce

1. Blend in blender.

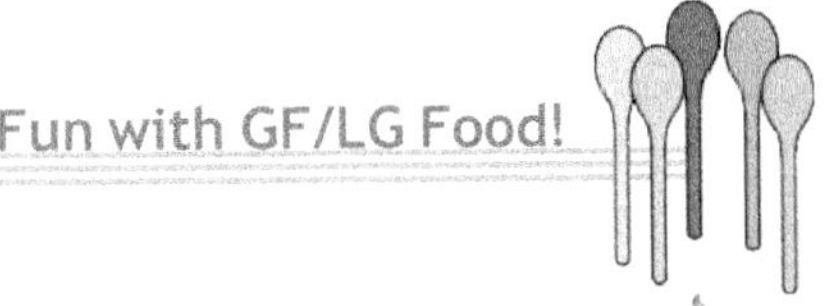

Variations

- Use a Fruit Topping made just exactly as you would make the Cherry Tart filling (p. 85), but use any kind of Fruit you like! I'd recommend Cherries, Strawberries, Blueberries or whatever fruit you love. They all go well with the Lemon.

Nut-sensitive people:

Replace the Walnuts with 1 cup of Amaranth Flour and increase Oil or Ghee to ¼ cup.

CHEESECAKE for Everyone!

For those who cannot eat dairy products, follow instructions for soaked cashews and coconut cream. Be sure to add salt if shown. This dessert has never been published before.

Special Note to Diabetics: I suppose you're wondering what this recipe is doing in a diabetic-friendly book? Well, one of the most famous diabetics of our time who has built many medical clinics was tested by three nurses after eating my cheesecake and his blood sugar was pronounced perfectly stable!

Makes: One 9" cheesecake

Ingredients:

Gluten-Free Walnut Crust

　　1 cup Organic Walnuts
　　1 tsp Cinnamon
　　1 Tbsp. Ghee
　　　　or 1 Tbsp. pur, virgin Coconut Oil
　　¼ tsp Celtic Sea Salt
　　　　or ¼ tsp Pink Himalayan Salt

1. Grind Walnuts until very fine, so they stick together
2. Mix in Cinnamon and Ghee or Coconut Oil.
3. Spread on bottom of 9" pie plate and press into pan. It's okay to cover just the bottom of the pan.

***Cashews:** Soak overnight or for 8 hours in pure Water. Drain and Measure, adding ¼ tsp Celtic Sea Salt or Pink Himalayan Salt.

Soaked Cashews may be kept refrigerated in Water for up to two days after soaking, then use must use or freeze them.

Filling

16 oz organic Cream Cheese
    or 16 oz soft Goat Cheese
    or 1½ cups soaked Cashews*
3 organic Eggs or Egg Replacer of choice
1 tsp organic Vanilla Extract
    or I tsp Vanilla Flavor (Celiacs may not tolerate extract)
3 drops organic Almond Extract
    or 3 drops Almond Flavor (Celiacs may not tolerate extract)
½ cup grade A organic Maple Syrup
½ tsp Sweet Leaf Stevia Extract, to taste
    or other form of Stevia, to taste
¼ cup organic Whipping Cream
    or creamy part of canned COconut Milk full-fat (not lite)
Juice of 1 small organic Lemon
Grated Peel of whole Lemon

1. Mix all ingredients with electric mixer, or mix well by hand until smooth.If using Cashews, you must use a blender. Blend until smooth.
2. Pour *gently* into unbaked Walnut Crust.
3. Place a pan with Water on bottom shelf of oven to keep Cheesecake from cracking.
4. Bake 2 hours at 200 °F. Check with toothpick to make sure center is done, even if slightly browned around edges. Or, bake it more slowly at 150-170 °F for about 3 hours or more and it will be wonderful!

Vegans: Replace the Ghee with cold-pressed virgin Coconut Oil.

Nut-sensitive people: Replace the Nut Meals with 1 cup Amaranth Flour and extra Oil—¼ cup or more if needed—to stick together.

GINGER-PUMPKIN CUSTARD PIE

Even though this recipe has no milk whatsoever, it is very rich and creamy if not over-baked.

Makes: One 9" pie

Ingredients:

Gluten-Free Crust
   2 Tbsp. Ghee
   ¼ tsp Celtic Sea Salt
      or ¼ tsp Pink Himalayan Salt
   1 Egg or Egg Replacer (add 1 Tbsp. Protein Powder if using Egg Replacer)
   ¼ cup Amaranth flour
   ¾ cup Pecan Meal (my favorite), finely ground
      —you may buy or grind your own in blender
      or Almond Meal/flour, finely ground

1. Melt Ghee or Coconut Oil on low heat. Melt in pie pan, if you want to wash fewer pans.
2. Mix Almond Meal and Flour, Salt and Egg or Egg Replacer with Protein Powder, if you use it, right in pie pan.

   Important Note: Mix until mixture clumps together, so the Oil spreads evenly and mixture presses well into pan and stays more firm.
3. Press into pie pan.

Filling

1 inch organic Ginger Root, sliced in about ¼ inch slices,
½ cup purified Water
3 organic or free-range Eggs
2 cups organic canned (check label to make sure it is
    100% Pumpkin and does not have other ingredients)
    or 2 cups organic fresh Pumpkin, baked and mashed
    or for natural sweetness, 1 cup Pumpkin and 1 cup Squash
    or Sweet Potato, baked and mashed
½ tsp Stevia of choice and
 1 Tbsp. Quinoa flour
½ tsp Celtic Sea Salt
    or ½ tsp Pink Himalayan Salt
1 tsp organic Cinnamon
½ tsp organic Nutmeg
½ tsp organic Allspice
1 tsp organic Vanilla Extract (optional)
    or 1 tsp vanilla flavor (Celiacs may not tolerate extract)
    or fresh organic Vanilla Bean

1. Blend in blender: Ginger Root, and Water, then pour into saucepan.
2. Bring Ginger mixture to a boil while doing next step.
3. In a separate heat-proof bowl, mix together remaining ingredients.
4. Add boiling Ginger mixture to dry ingredients and pour into 9" pie shell.
5. Bake 400 °F for 15 minutes (375 °F for 30 minutes). Check. Best if not too firm.

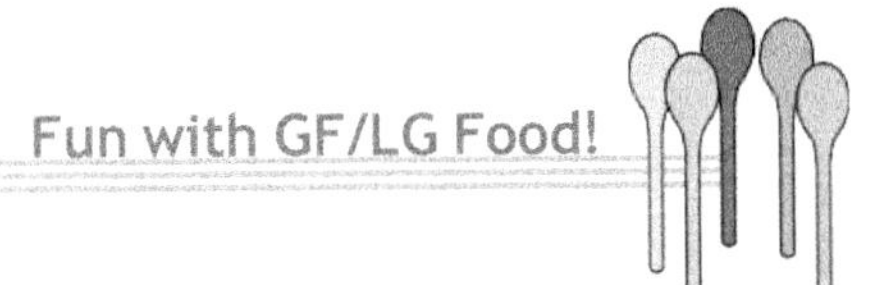

Variations

- Replace Mint with organic Cherry Flavoring and ½ cup chopped organic Sweet Cherries, fresh or frozen.
- Replace Mint with organic Orange Flavoring and 1 Tbsp. Orange Zest.
- For a classic Brownie: replace Mint with ½ cup toasted organic Walnuts.
- If you are a hard-core chocolate-lover, try straight organic, non-sweetened Cocoa Powder or organic Cacao Nibs (health food store) in place of Carob Powder, or use half Carob Powder and half Cacao, or add unsweetened Dark Chocolate Chips.

Vegans: Replace Egg with Egg Substitute of choice.

Dairy-sensitive people: Replace Ghee with organic virgin Coconut Oil.

Nut-sensitive people: Replace Almond Meal with a combination of Quinoa and Amaranth Flours.

Golden Chalice
CAROB MINT BROWNIES

From our "I Can't Believe it's Not Chocolate" collection—if you don't tell your guests, they may never know!

Makes: one 8" x 8" pan

Ingredients:
- ½ cup organic Ghee (clarified Butter)
  - or I stick organic Butter
  - ½ cup organic Carob Powder
- ¼ cup roasted organic Chicory Root (provides more chocolatey flavor), finely ground in coffee-grinder
- 1 tsp organic Vanilla Extract
  - or 1 tsp Vanilla Flavor (Celiacs may not tolerate extract)
- 1 tsp organic Peppermint Extract
  - or 1 tsp Peppermint Flavor (Celiacs may not tolerate extract)
  - 2 organic or free-range Eggs
- 1 cup organic Almond Meal
- 1 tsp Baking Powder
- ½ tsp Celtic Sea Salt
  - or ½ tsp Pink Himalayan Salt

1. Preheat oven to 350 °F.
2. Melt Ghee or Oil in baking dish (8" x 8") to save dish washing.
3. Stir in Carob Powder, Chicory, Extracts, Eggs.
4. Mix together and add to above mixture: Almond Meal or Flour, Baking Powder and Salt.
5. Bake 25-30 minutes. Will be fudge-like when cooled if not over-baked. Top should almost bounce back when touched. Cover immediately for more fudge-like texture.

Variations

- Add 1 whole organic Orange Peel, grated (on large grate if you're in a hurry or like the robust flavor) If you don't like Orange, leave it out.
- Add 1 tsp organic Cinnamon instead of Orange for a unique twist.
- Add ¼ to ½ cup organic shredded, unsweetened Coconut instead of or in addition to Orange flavor.
- Add about 1 cup combined organic Raisins and Sunflower Seeds.

Nut-sensitive people: In place of organic cream or Sweet Cashew Cream in any recipe, try Coconut Milk, found in health food and Asian stores. Use the creamy part which has risen to the top of the can. You can flavor and sweeten it to taste the same way you would Sweet Cashew Cream.

BANANA-ORANGE NUT (or not) BREAD

Thinking of fruit cake gifts for the holidays? Why not make it real fruit that doesn't need added sweetener, just nature's own. This is a rich, warm dessert to warm the heart. Can be used as cake, too, with a rich Cream Cheese Frosting (p. 79), Sweet Cashew Cream (p. 41 or 80), or Coconut Milk (thick part)

Makes: 2 loaves or one 9" cake

Ingredients:

3 large-size ripe organic Bananas
    or 4 medium/5 small ripe organic Bananas
1 organic or free-range Egg
½ tsp Stevia (or more to taste)
1 stick softened organic Butter or Ghee (clarified Butter)
    or ½ cup virgin organic Coconut Oil
    —I often combine them and use ¼ cup each
1 ½ cups Almond Meal Flour
2 Tbsps. Protein Powder (binds better)
½ cup organic Quinoa or Amaranth Flour or ½ cup combination of these Flours
1 tsp aluminum-free Baking Soda (health food store)
1 tsp Celtic Sea Salt
    or 1 tsp Pink Himalayan Salt
½ to 1 cup chopped organic Walnuts or Pecans (optional)
Flavorings of choice (see variations)

1. Mash Bananas in a large bowl. Melt Ghee, Butter or Oil.
2. Beat in Egg, Stevia and melted Butter or Oil.
3. Mix together: Almond Meal and/or Flours, Baking Soda, Salt.
4. Add Flour mixture to Banana mixture, along with your choice of flavorings.
5. Bake in two small bread pans, a bundt pan or 9" cake pan at 350 °F for ½-¾ hour or more. Wait until top starts to get firm, glossy and golden and then press down gently with your finger. If it bounces back, it's done. Don't let it get too brown.
6. After it cools for about ½ hour, cover or eat.

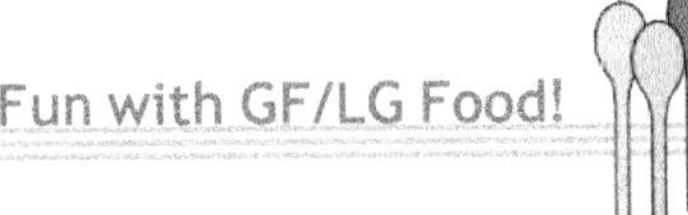

Variations

- Instead of Mangos, use 1 cup organic, unsweetened or raw Strawberries (frozen is just fine or thawed with Juice).
- Instead of Mangos, use 1 cup organic, unsweetened Peaches, same instructions as for Strawberries.
- Instead of Mangos, use 1 cup organic, unsweetened Blueberries, follow same instructions as for Strawberries. For an extra special treat, fold in ½ cup coarsely chopped pieces of Cheesecake for Everyone! (p. 92) at the very end, after whipping Blueberry Mixture. Voila! You now have Blueberry Cheesecake Ice Cream!

MANGO FROZEN MOUSSE

This can be served as a very rich mousse as well.

Serves: Four to eight people

Ingredients:

1 medium or large ripe organic Mango
1 cup Whipping Cream
    or 1 cup Sweet Cashew Cream (p. 41 or 80)
    or 1 pint (1 can) full-fat Coconut Milk
2 tsp organic Vanilla Extract
    or 2 tsp Vanilla Flavor (Celiacs may not tolerate extract)

1. Blend in blender Mango, 2 Tbsp. or more Whipping Cream, Cashew Cream or Coconut Milk. Use as much Cream or Milk as needed to make blender run, but no more. If using Cashew Cream or Coconut Milk, just blend it all with the Mango and go to step 5.
2. In mixing bowl, whip remaining Cream and Extract or Flavoring.
3. Beat until it looks like soft Whipping Cream (not too stiff or hard).
4. Blend in Mango Mixture.
5. Taste to see if any Stevia or other sweetener is needed. Freeze, if you can wait that long to eat it! Or eat it as Mousse .. yum.

   Important Note: Defrost for 15-30 minutes in order to have this ice cream soft enough to enjoy. The texture will be too icy otherwise. Or, if you're dedicated to true ice cream texture, take out of freezer every half hour for 2 hours, stir with a fork, then return to freezer.

Variations

- Frontier Organics makes a great Coffee Flavor. Use 1 Tbsp. in place of the Carob Powder and Peppermint.
- Replace chicory and carob with finely ground unsweetened organic Coconut (grind in dedicated coffee grinder) and add 2 tsp organic Coconut Extract or Flavor.
- Replace Carob and Chicory with 1 Tbsp. organic Lemon or Orange Zest and 1 tsp organic Lemon or Orange Extract or Flavor.
- Go Nuts! Try whatever flavorings you like. Add Nuts. Make basic Vanilla (just use the Whipped Cream recipe and freeze it!) Play with Sauces. Try the variations on the Banana-Orange Sauce (p. 43, 56 or 83). Or purchase organic Sauces made just from Fruit—I do not recommend those with high-fructose Corn Syrup. Always check labels and taste a small amount.)

I Can't Believe it's Not Chocolate CAROB-MINT FROZEN MOUSSE

Very rich, but very easy and quick, this can be served as a Mousse as well, without freezing.

Serves: Four to eight people

Ingredients:
- ½ pint (1 cup) organic Whipping Cream
  - or 1 cup Sweet Cashew Cream (p. 41 or 80)
  - or 1 pint (1 can) full-fat Coconut Milk
- 2 tsp organic Vanilla Extract
  - or 2 tsp Vanilla Flavor (Celiacs may not tolerate extract)
- ½ tsp organic Peppermint Extract
  - or ½ tsp Peppermint Flavor (Celiacs may not tolerate extract)
- 2 Tbsp. organic (if possible) Carob powder
- 1 Tbsp. organic roasted Chicory Root finely ground in coffee grinder
- 1 Tbsp. organic pure Maple Syrup
- ¼ tsp Sweet Leaf Stevia, to taste
  - or other form of Stevia, to taste

1. In large mixing bowl, mix all ingredients and whip until firm. Beat until it looks like soft Whipping Cream (not too stiff or hard). No need to whip if using Coconut Milk.
2. Freeze, if you can wait that long to eat it! Or eat some first as Mousse.

Important Note: Defrost for 15-30 minutes in order to have this ice cream soft enough to enjoy. The texture will be too icy otherwise. Or, if you're dedicated to true ice cream texture, take out of freezer every half hour for 2 hours, stir with a fork, then return to freezer.

Success Secret: To make carob taste more like chocolate, you can use something bitter (like the roasted chicory) and something flavorful (like the mint, cherry or orange). Find chicory root online or call Present Moment Herb Shop in Minneapolis, MN, 612-824-3157.

Variations

- For a creamier version: Add 2 Tbsp. or more Organic Cream, Yogurt, or Coconut Milk (creamy!) to taste.
- For a sweeter version: Add Green Leaf Ground Stevia, to taste.
- For other flavors: Add Mint Extract, Orange, Cherry, Almond, etc., to taste.

Vegans: Replace Gelatin with agar-agar (see package directions).

People with sensitivities: Aveena Originals has a protein powder with no gluten, milk, soy, corn or brown rice (call 800-207-2239).

CAROB-MOCHA HIGH PROTEIN SHAKE

Want a shake, but want it to be nutritious? Here you go! This takes some prep work, but you can keep the prep stuff in fridge for a few days till ready. The Shake keeps well, too.

Serves: This recipe is measured in "per person" amounts.

Ingredients—adjust measurements to personal taste—these are approximate:

10-20 Soaked, germinated Almonds
   (soaked 16 hours in purified Water, rinsed every 8 hours, then refrigerated—use within 2 days)
¼ cup Unflavored Gelatin,
   mixed with ½ the recommended boiling Water and refrigerated to use as needed. To speed up the process, mix gelatin and melt with just a little boiling Water, then add cool Water)
¼ cup Soaked Raisins and some of the Water
   (Soak Raisins in jar, covering them with Water well over the top of the Raisins—but less than twice as much Water as Raisins)
1 Tbsp. of your favorite Protein
Powder 1 Tbsp. roasted organic Carob
powder 1 tsp ground roasted Chicory
Root
   finely ground in coffee grinder
1 tsp Vanilla Extract
   or 1 tsp Vanilla Flavor (Celiacs may not tolerate extract)
Dash Celtic Sea Salt, to taste
   or dash Pink Himalayan Salt, to taste
¼ to ½ cup of Water to allow blender to work
   —add more if needed to personal taste

1. Blend all ingredients in blender and enjoy!

Chapter 6
Breads, Snacks and Light Meals for the Road

I know it's hard at times to think of what travels well and will be satisfying. I do a lot of traveling and actually bring a week's worth of food in a cooler and let hotel management know I need a refrigerator. The following ideas may help you in this day and age, they have certainly helped me.

Success Secret: If your bread comes out too moist, as mine sometimes does, this firms it up. Put the bread back in the oven after turning it off and let the loaf dry out. Or, if later (after refrigerating bread), heat the oven to 300 °F and place bread in oven on sheet or in pan and let it dry out. Check in 20 minutes or sooner if the loaf is already well done. If not dry enough, leave in oven and check every 10 minutes.

A big Thank You goes to Dr. Sondra Traylor, D.C., N.D., L.Ac. for taking the time and love to develop a basic recipe. It was easy to adapt into a flavorful recipe 'most anyone will like. I do my own spin on it and you can, too. The bottom line is; do whatever works!

Breads

SPROUTED SOUFFLÉ FLATBREAD

Rich and flavorful, this bread has become a staple in my special diet. It very well may do so for you, too. It fills me up when I'm still hungry and don't have other choices to eat right then. Flatbread can be savory or a dessert, depending on how you dress it up. Great snack food!

I know the title sounds like an oxymoron. It is flatbread because it doesn't rise, and it's like soufflé because of all the eggs, which hold it together without the gluten! The flavor is wonderful*. Use the New Twists for easy-to-travel-with treats.

Makes: 10 large-enough-to-toast pieces of bread

Ingredients:
- 1 cup sprouted organic gluten-free Grains, Nuts and/or Seeds and/or Beans of choice (p. 13)
- ¼ cup high heat Oil, such as:
    organic Oil of Choice, high heat Sunflower Oil
    or cold-pressed, virgin Coconut Oil, melted
- ½ tsp or more Celtic Sea Salt, to taste
    or ½ tsp or more Pink Himalayan Salt, to taste
- 2 large organic Eggs
- ½ Apple, cut in slices
- ¼ tsp Sweet Leaf Stevia, to taste
    or other form of Stevia, to taste
- 1 heaping tsp Arrowroot Powder

1. Oil a 13" x 9" x 2" pan or cookie sheet. Preheat oven to 350 °F.
2. Blend all ingredients in blender until smooth. If you like a heartier texture, do not blend as much.
3. Pour into pan, smooth out to even height and bake for 20-30 minutes or until brown. Don't worry if bubbles appear, or if the entire top raises up, it will go back down after it's done. This is why I call it Soufflé Bread!

4. Let cool and cut into pieces the size you like. Make sure they are long enough to get out of the toaster, or just turn your toaster upside down to release bread (I've had to do that when I cut them too small—live and learn).

5. Turn Bread bottom side up to spread Butter or other Spreads on it. It will hold better.

NEW TWISTS ON SPROUTED SOUFFLÉ FLATBREAD

There are so many wonderful ways to enjoy this treat. Use your imagination to come up with your own new twists!

- **Rosemary Bread**—Add tsp organic dried Rosemary to blender. Use ½ the sweetener.
- **Dill Bread**—Add 1 tsp organic dried Dill Weed to blender. Use ½ the sweetener.
- **Onion or Onion-Dill Bread**—Add ½ cup chopped Onion to top of uncooked Bread in pan and then put in oven. For Onion-Dill Bread, just add 1 tsp organic dried Dill Weed to blender. Use ½ the sweetener.
- **Cinnamon-Raisin Bread**—You can add before blending or stir Raisins in after blending if you prefer your Raisins whole. Add ½ tsp Sweet Leaf Stevia for a sweeter Bread.
- **Simple, Nutritious Carrot Cake**—Add ½ cup more Carrots in the blender, ½ tsp Sweet Leaf Stevia. Add to blended mixture, but do not blend again: Raisins and Carrot-Cake Spices (p. 78) for a Carrot Cake with healthy, sprouted Grains and Seeds!
- **Hide Your Vegetables Bread**—Add whatever Vegetables you like, but choose more dense Root Vegetables and Squash family or Legumes and stay away from more Watery ones like Cucumber.
- **Cheesy Bread**—Stir in after blending: ½ cup shredded organic Cheese of choice—or sprinkle on top just before removing from oven.
- **Chili Bread**—Stir in after blending: 1 Tbsp. or more (based on your hot-button) chopped Chili Peppers, canned Jalapeño Peppers and organic, cooked Black Beans.

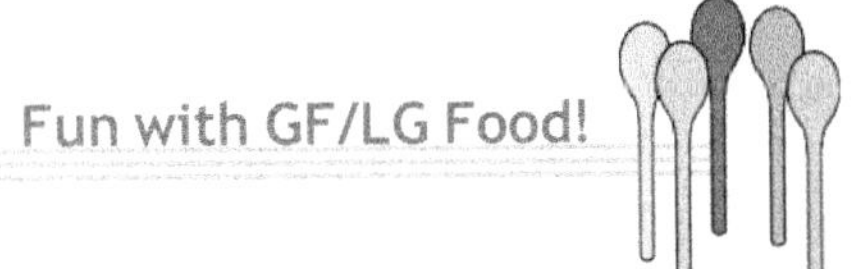

SROUTED GRAINS AND SEEDS
FOR BREAD

Makes: About 1 cup, depending on combination chosen

Ingredients:

½ cup combined Grains, Seeds, Beans and/or Nuts, if you can eat them. It takes less time to sprout the following: Quinoa, Amaranth, Sesame and Sunflower seeds, Red Lentils and Wild Rice...and I know that combination works for the bread)

1. Place Grains, Seeds, Beans and/or Nuts into pint or larger jar.
2. Fill with Water and let soak overnight or all day.
3. Rinse thoroughly. You can soak for a total of 24 hours, rinsing at least once during that time. If you use larger Grains, Nuts and Beans, soak for 24 hours.

Success Secret: I recommend using nonmetal pans, such as ceramic or glass, like Pyrex, for baking or cooking (no metallic flavor!), unless you can afford pure titanium cookware. (Check your local upscale kitchen store or online.) Many health practitioners warn against heavy metal toxicity, so I stay away from using metal cookware since it is being heated with the food.

Variations

- Add and blend in: 1 Tbsp. or more chopped Chili Peppers (depending on your hot-button), canned Jalapeño Peppers and organic, cooked Black Beans.
- Add and blend in: shredded organic Cheese of any kind (Raw Milk Goat Cheese, Vegan Almond Cheese, etc.), or sprinkle on top just before removing from oven.

Nut-sensitive people:

Replace Almond Meal with Amaranth Flour.

BLUE CORNBREAD

Here's an alternate to high-glycemic fare for those who can eat corn and would like a little of the flavor with a lower-glycemic content. This recipe uses very little cornmeal. Blue cornmeal has a higher protein level than yellow or white varieties.

Makes: 8" x 8" pan

Ingredients:
- ½ cup organic Blue Cornmeal
- ½ cup organic Quinoa flour
    - or ½ cup organic Quinoa soaked, to make moister bread
- 1 cup organic Almond Meal
- I tsp aluminum-free baking powder
- ½ tsp Celtic Sea Salt
    - or ½ tsp Pink Himalayan Salt
- 1 organic egg
- 1 cup purified Water or any kind of Milk or Yogurt
- ½ cup virgin Coconut Oil
    - or ½ cup Oil of Choice (higher flash-point)
- ½ tsp Sweet Leaf Stevia, to taste
    - or other form of Stevia, to taste

1. Preheat oven to 375 °F. Blend together Cornmeal, Flours, Baking Powder and Salt.
2. Add and blend in the Egg, Water, Oil and Stevia.
3. Use a 8" x 8" pan or muffin tins and bake for 20-25 minutes or until done.

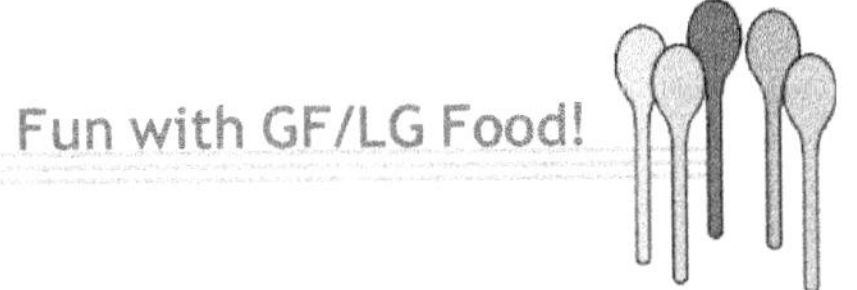

INSTANT FRENCH TOAST

Serves: This recipe is measured in "per person" amounts.

Ingredients per person:
Sprouted Soufflé Flatbread
Cinnamon, to taste

1. Simply sprinkle Cinnamon on Flatbread before traveling or bring Cinnamon along to sprinkle it on fresh.

Variation
- Bring along Fruit Spread—try the variations on Banana-Orange Sauce (p. 43, 56 or 83)—and/or Almond Butter.

Variations

- Bring Veggie Sticks (p. 111) of sliced Vegetables such as organic Carrot, Celery, Zucchini, Cabbage or Bok Choy slices for dipping.
- Make sandwiches out of Sprouted Soufflé Flatbread by turning bread bottom-side-up, to better hold dressings and other sandwich ingredients.
- Bring Avocado with knife or Guacamole (p. 9) sprinkled generously with Lemon Juice to keep it from getting brown.

Light Meals for the Road

TRAVEL SPREADS—Version 1

1. Bring along your favorite savory rendition of the Sprouted Souffle Flatbread (p. 102) in a container and/or gluten-free Chips or Crackers of choice if you want to splurge. Bring several pieces per person. Use ¼ cup per person of any of the Spreads in chapter 1, such as Hummus, Sunflower Pate or Bean Dip in travel container. Be sure to carry in cooler.
2. Bring a plastic knife and spoon for spreading spreads. You may also want to bring along small reusable plates or sturdy napkins.

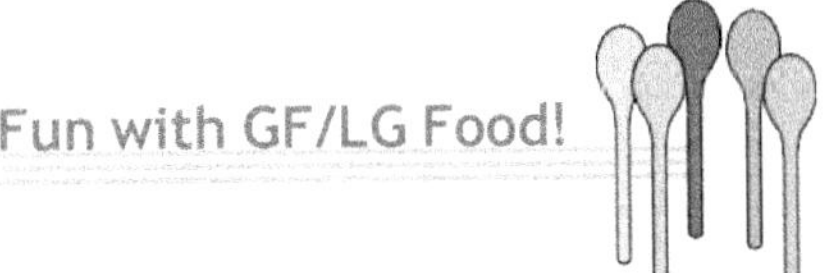

Variations

- Instead of Bread or Crackers, slice organic Apples to use as base for Nut Butters.
- Bring organic Chevre (soft Goat Cheese) or other Cheese of your choice to spread on Sprouted Soufflé Flatbread or Apples.
- Make sandwiches out of Sprouted Soufflé Flatbread by turning bread bottom-side-up, to better hold dressings and other sandwich ingredients.

TRAVEL SPREADS—Version 2

1. Pack your favorite sweet or neutral rendition of the Sprouted Souffle Flatbread (p. 102) in a container and/or gluten-free Chips or Crackers of choice if you want to splurge. Bring several pieces per person.
2. Bring ¼ cup per person of any of your favorite Nut Butters or Fruit Spreads or leftover Fruit Sauce—try the variations on Banana-Orange Sauce (p. 43, 56 or 83). You can make a jam by simply cooking a little more Water out of the sauce.
3. Bring a plastic knife and spoon for spreading spreads. You may also want to bring along small reusable plates or sturdy napkins.

For Shorter Trips

ROASTED OR SPROUTED NUTS AND SEEDS

1. Tamari-flavored Roasted Nuts and/or Seeds (p. 12).
2. Sprouted Nuts and/or Seeds (p. 13).

HARD BOILED EGGS

High-protein snack.

1. Boil two organic Eggs per person, peel Eggs, place in travel container and Salt. Be sure to carry in cooler.
2. Slice fun and colorful Veggies like organic Red Bell Pepper, Carrots and Celery. Place in travel container and cooler.

TRUFFLES

1. Coconut or Carob-Walnut Truffles (p. 89) travel great and are filling.

CINNAMON APPLES

1. Slice organic Apples in thin slices.
2. Sprinkle with organic, freshly ground Cinnamon. If you want the Cinnamon more evenly distributed, shake in jar or travel container.

Credit for this incredibly tasty, naturally sweet treat goes to my friend Deb Z. Thank you, Deb!

Variation
- For spiced apple cider flavor, simply toss in a pinch of ground Cloves with the Cinnamon before you shake the jar.

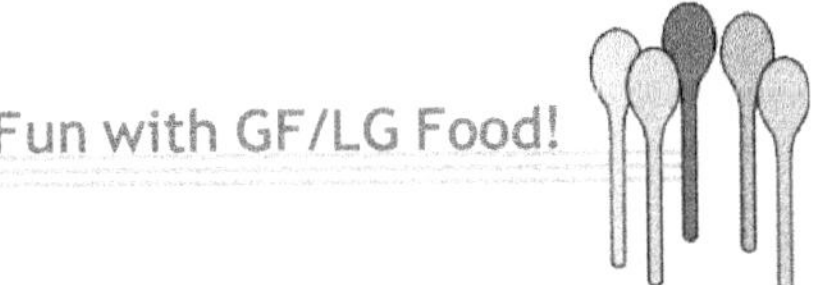

For Longer Trips

1. Bring cooked organic Meat, Chicken, sliced Turkey, wild-caught Salmon (not as fishy smelling as other types of fish, but canned Tuna or Sardines can work if you remember can-opener!), hard-boiled Eggs, sprouted Nuts and Seeds and dry Nuts and Seeds to sprout in your hotel room or kitchen.
2. Bring small containers of your own Salad Dressing (see House Dressing p. 34) or purchase when you arrive.
3. Buy organic Salad mix when you get there. Most grocery stores have it now.
4. Bring a few essential Herbs or Spices so you can play with your food. For example, you can slice Apples and sprinkle with Cinnamon.

Success Secret: In hotels I use the guest drinking glasses to sprout small amounts of nuts or seeds overnight. I also heat hard boiled eggs and cooked bacon by filling the ice bucket with really hot water and putting my container in it.

Variation

- To be creative, try raw Root Vegetables like Turnips sliced raw. Radishes and other Veggies do well. Zucchini and Italian Yellow Squash may not last as long, but work for a day or two.

VEGGIE STICKS

The obvious, but least remembered. Wonderful to have when you can't get organic salad, these last for days in a good cooler.

Serves: This recipe is measured in "per person" amounts.

Ingredients per person:
Organic Carrots
Organic Celery
Organic Red Cabbage
Organic Bok Choy
Organic Broccoli Stems
Organic Sugar Snap Peas

1. Slice in any way you like for snacks. Pack in green veggie bags to last longer (ask your health food store)

Success Secret: When staying in motels, I use their ice to replace my own or I ask for a refrigerator for "medical reasons" which is all they understand when you have special health needs.

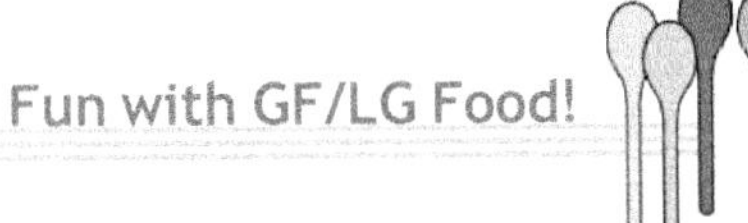

- Add chopped very ripe organic tropical Fruits such as Mango, Papaya, fresh or dried organic Coconut. For more flavor, grind coconut in food processor or dedicated coffee grinder.
- Instead of (or in addition to) Banana add 1 tsp roasted organic Carob Powder, ¼ tsp roasted Chicory Root, finely ground in coffee grinder, and ¼ tsp Almond Extract or Flavor. Optional: Also add 1 Tbsp. Almond Butter.
- Replace Banana with chopped fruit such as Peach, Strawberry, Cherry, Blueberry. Yum!
- Replace Bananas with Toasted Pecans (p. 12) Add ½ tsp organic Maple Flavor.
- Replace Banana with ¼ to ½ organic Lemon or Orange Zest. (I keep fresh organic Zest in small containers in refrigerator for a week or more and are fine!)

Vegans and dairy-sensitive people: Replace the Yogurt with Coconut Milk. Use top, creamy layer for a thicker texture. Blend if using Protein Powder or other thickener.

HI-PROTEIN YOGURT PUDDING

If you like smooth and creamy treats, this truly instant pudding is for you, and it travels well, too!

Serves: This recipe is measured in "per person" amounts.

Ingredients per person:
    ½ cup plain organic Goat Yogurt
        or ½ cup whole Milk Yogurt (if you can find it!)
    1 Tbsp. unsweetened Protein Powder of choice (optional)
    2 Tbsp. sprouted organic Almonds or Seeds
    ½ tsp organic Vanilla Extract
        or ½ tsp Vanilla Flavor (Celiacs may not tolerate extract)
    ¼ tsp Sweet Leaf Stevia, to taste
        or other form of Stevia, to taste
    ½ organic Banana

1. Place yogurt in bowl or travel container.
2. Chop Banana into very small pieces and blend into yogurt with rest of ingredients.
3. Chop Almonds and garnish top of Pudding with them.

Variations

Success Secret: Your turn! What else can you come up with? (Oh yeah, I forgot about coconut pudding, but I bet you can figure it out by now...coconut and coconut extract or coconut flavor!)

Bonus Section

Eating In Restaurants

First of all, I must make a disclaimer: If you have Celiac disease, you must check with your doctor to see if you can even eat in restaurants at all, since the littlest piece of gluten flour or crumb that gets into your food, as you may know by now unless you are new to this disease, will affect your health negatively.

Restaurant dining has been a challenge for me, having been vegetarian for awhile and also not wanting to eat wheat or sugar! I found that even substitutes like honey did me in. I'd be flattened by too much of any grain or starch. My low blood sugar was talking to me!

Also, I found I actually liked vegetables! And as my friend Jocelyn says, "Vegetables are our friends." It's so true. How else are we going to improve our health, but with our food? There is no better way to assure a steady stream of good nutrients.

But it was so hard to get low-starch veggies in most restaurants. Restaurants can be a bear, unless it was mine, ***The Golden Chalice,*** and unfortunately, it's gone...but lucky you! Now you don't need them with all this travel food.

I rarely eat in restaurants anymore because my own food, healthy as it is, actually tastes better than almost anything I can eat out. You'll get to feel the same way, I have no doubt, if you truly use the best quality ingredients, as I recommend.

There is one exception to this generality: Truly gourmet restaurants. Since I don't eat out that often, and you probably don't either, you can spend more on eating out. It's like I read years ago in Dress for Success "...Pay twice as much and buy half as many" and they last longer, too...Same with a really, really fine meal. You'll probably never forget it. So:

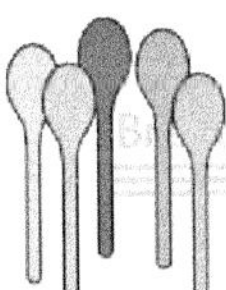

Tip # 1— Eat in very fine, high quality restaurants. Eat out half as much and—now don't flinch here—pay twice as much!! Yes, you can do it, just save what you'd spend now on later. Or, if you have to, save your pennies and nickels and dimes and even quarters and put them in a jar and count them at the end of two months and you will likely be able to go to a very fine restaurant. There, you will be more assured of finer care.

Tip #2—Use the menu as a base to see what they have in the kitchen but tell the server exactly what you want and how you want it done. You don't even need to say you have some disease or other, because if you say it with confidence they'll just think you are an obscure television star they've never seen. Really, though, if you have Celiac disease you should let them know you are gluten-sensitive and to be very cautious about what goes into your food. Top chefs should take good care of you.

Tip # 3—Know this: Bored chefs love to make special meals for people. So go when you know it won't be busy, Sunday or Monday nights, or early, as soon as they open for dinner at 5 or 5:30 p.m.

Tip # 4—Vegetables are our friends. Order mostly vegetables made fresh, like salad, grilled vegetables, etc. And "grill" the servers over what's in the soup. If they hem and haw, get the manager or chef out to your table. They will usually comply in a fancy restaurant and you will feel very special.

Tip # 5—Tell them to 86 the bread. Or more nicely put, "I/ we don't eat bread, so please don't bring it to the table." If others at the table want bread, and you are really hungry, ask if you can order some soup, salad or appetizer right away so you can eat it while everyone else munches on their intestinal dry-wall.

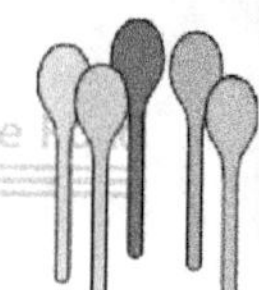

Tip # 6—Ideas for simple meals:

- Find a special salad you like and simply have them add grilled fish, chicken, beef of your choice or cheese and nuts for vegetarians and toasted nuts/seeds for vegans.
- Whatever delicious-looking main course they have can be dressed up with your choice of vegetables and salad.
- If a particular sauce, such as an Italian sauce (no chance of gluten-containing flour in it—but ask anyway) looks good to you, ask for it on your meat or fish or veggies, or whatever, but make sure of the ingredients first.
- If a sandwich appeals to you from the menu, even if it's a hamburger (albeit a high-class hamburger), ask to have it served exactly as is, even topped with the pesto-mayo, sauces or whatever. Just ask to have it made without the bun or bread. Make sure that if they accidentally put it on the bread they make it over it for you!!
- You can also request a lettuce wrap of the sandwich. If they are clueless, tell them to cut the innards (okay, better say ingredients) of the sandwich into smaller bits and plop them (place them sounds better, on second thought) on the lettuce or if they happen to have Chinese cabbage, that works well, too. The leaf can be left as is or rolled and held in place with a toothpick.

Tip # 7—Tell them that for dessert you would like some fresh fruit. See what's on the dessert menu and they will likely have it. Mango is often available because it's a popular ingredient in chi-chi salsas, etc. Use your best detective nose when snooping through the menu.

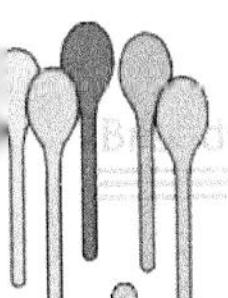

Mexican Cuisine

Authentic Mexican food has very little wheat/cheese/milk—think fish Vera Cruz, fajitas, real tamales, huevos rancheros, etc.

Tips for gluten and dairy sensitive people:

- Make sure Mexican sauces or salsas are "sin trigo" or "sin gluten" (wheat-free or gluten-free).
- Many authentic Mexican meals do not automatically come with flour tortillas. You can decline them or request corn tortillas instead.
- Some not-so-authentic Mexican restaurants add other ingredients (such as wheat) to corn tortillas or fry corn chips in oil that was used to fry gluten-containing foods (such as chimichangas). Be sure to ask.
- If the restaurant has milk products on the menu for gringos, just request no cheese ("no queso") or no milk ("no leche") in your food.

Contributed by my brilliant book-formatting and graphic artist, Sunni Bradshaw.

More Tricks for Eating in Restaurants

Choose Asian cuisine whenever possible.
Here you can get yummy, stir-fried, but not over-cooked veggies with or without meat. Here are the tips:

Be sure to ask for a sauce without sugar, cornstarch or MSG. Keep in mind that many soy sauces are made with wheat. Tell them to hold the rice.

If you order soup, be sure it's made without sugar. In many restaurants, it will already have MSG. For more protein, ask them to add nuts if you can eat them. Hold the peanuts, which tend toward mold.

If your body likes soy, ask for tofu, which they usually have. An alternative idea: Ask for egg stir-fried into your vegetables, similar to fried rice, but without the rice. (Rice is the highest glycemic grain!).

Vegans, ask for nuts and seeds (for extra protein) and vegetarians, ask for cheese, eggs and/or nuts and seeds.

Celiacs, ask for no sauce and bring your own small bottle of Braggs Liquid Amino Acids or wheat-free soy sauce or wheat-free tamari. You can make your own meal of sauteed veggies and meats/fish/nuts.

Be sure to send the chef your compliments.

Appendix A
Vegetables and Ingredients I Don't Use and Why

I learned this information from various health practitioners, researchers in health and experts in digestion. I am not a doctor—so once again, please talk with your doctor about any doubts or concerns about leaving these ingredients out of your diet.

Brown Rice: As a low glycemic grain, in general, brown rice is slow to digest unless cooked very slowly, on low heat, over a long period of time. Even then it still disagrees with many people's digestive systems. Brown basmati rice is better. White whole-grain basmati rice is best—though we stay away from very starchy, high carbohydrate foods for optimum health and blood-sugar balance for most people.

Broccoli Tops (Florets), Cauliflower, Head Lettuce, Brussels Sprouts: All are hybrids, very difficult to digest unless cooked well, which I do not do to maintain some good digestive enzymes and more life-giving qualities. Contains digestive- inhibiting enzymes, so in raw form, difficult to digest. Broccoli stems have all the nutrients! These are used with delight.

Bread: Filler food that can create problems in the intestines if not whole grain or 100% sprouted. *Celiacs: sprouted wheat is not gluten free.* Bread is also very high in complex carbohydrates which most people need very little of and may be healthier without. You will find a recipe on p. 102 for a sprouted bread that is much higher in nutrients, easier to digest and has no flour whatsoever, no yeast, no baking soda or baking powder and is delicious!

Canola Oil or Soy Oil: Processing of these oils can create rancidity (free radical issue) because they are exposed to high heat during processing. Deodorizing agents and chemicals used during extraction cannot be sufficiently removed. Not very digestible.

Important Note: Olive oil should *not* be used for cooking, as it has a very low flash point, so it turns rancid quickly.

Carbonated Beverages: If combined with sugars, carbonation forces higher intake of sugars into the cells. Makes digestion more difficult in general. Natural carbonation, such as in Pelligrino water may be okay, carbonated Water in general is okay for occasional use.

Chocolate, Caffeine, Alcohol: All are addictive substances, all are hard on the liver, which cleanses the blood.

Gluten Flours: I use gluten-free and grains (they are really not grains, but seeds) such as amaranth and quinoa. Unfortunately, millet seems to be cross-contaminated with gluten-containing grains now. (Celiacs can get very ill with any gluten). Those of us interested in maintaining better health, digestion eliminate or reduce gluten-containing grains in our diets.

Grains in General: Imagine you are a primitive man and woman trying to eke out a meager meal from the environment, in the cold at that, what would you go for first? Look around you—especially in spring, fall and summer—you see mostly green, right? That's what we should be focusing on the most: vegetables!

Next, you might have killed an animal, even small. Berries in spring, nuts and seeds in fall, root vegetables for winter. You would learn how to store these, plus squash and some fruit. But you would have to laboriously crack open each nut and seed. Do you think you would then have the time or inclination to peel the chaff from each grain? Of course you would figure it out, as the Native Americans did, how to beat the chaff off, but how much grain could you really eat?

Grains are not something our bodies need in any quantity at all. Some people, like myself, eat none at all unless the grains are sprouted or on very special occasions. Even then, my body rebels. Quinoa and amaranth, among some others of like origin, are really seeds, not grains, and are much easier on us. See Appendix B.

Millet: Millet is a wonderful high protein grain in its natural state, but it is often cross-contaminated, so I don't recommend it to Celiacs or Diabetics in case they may have Celiac disease (getting to be more common in Type I diabetes)

Most Mushrooms: Usually grown in animal fertilizer and need to be very well cleansed and soaked in peroxide to kill probable parasites. I use shitake mushrooms (should be grown on trees), which have more health benefits.

Raw Nuts or Seeds: I find that Nuts and Seeds, roasted or sprouted, have digestive inhibitors so they will not sprout until they are in Water (nature thus assures their proper growth). These affect our digestion. So my recipes are either sprouted or roasted (kills digestive inhibiting enzymes.)

Peanuts or Peanut Oil: Usually contains mold that naturally grows on peanuts. Peanuts have a tendency toward mold. During processing, these molds can be transferred into the oil. Chemical agents used in processing may also remain in oil.

Refined Sugar, Honey: Very concentrated sweet and may pull minerals from the body. Not very good for most people. Many people find they are much healthier and more energetic without these. My desserts are sweetened with combinations

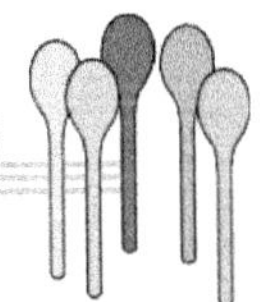

of whole fruits (not juice, which often contains concentrates loaded with high-fructose corn syrup) and sweet leaf stevia. Rarely I include a small amount of pure Maple Syrup with high-protein desserts like cheesecake.

Soy Products: Except for amino acids extracted from soy, such as in soy sauce or Braggs Liquid Amino Acids, soy is a protein that's very difficult to digest…the human digestive system does not have the capacity to break down the long chain amino acids of soy unless raised on it, such as Asians may be. Estrogen can increase from the ingestion of soy products. Though elevated estrogen levels may help some people, this can be non-beneficial for others and even may lead to disease. Most soy is processed with chemicals to which some people are sensitive. Many soy sauces contain also wheat.

Vinegar: Kills enzymes necessary for digestion—but can be used for marinades which are then cooked—if raw, use unfiltered apple cider vinegar.

Important Note: You'll notice non-stick pans are not recommended unless naturally non-stick titanium because they peel off and are not known for sure to be safe for your health.

Appendix B
Specific Ingredients
I Suggest In Recipes
and Why

I learned information from various health practitioners, researchers in health and experts in digestion. I am not a doctor. So once again, please discuss with your doctor any doubts or concerns about including these ingredients in your diet.

Broccoli Spears: Most of the nutrients in broccoli are in the stem. See Appendix A for reasons we don't use tops.

Braggs Liquid Amino Acids: I recommend this product because there is really no other to use for vegan meals that have flavor, are gluten-free and are easy to digest. While it is made with soy protein, it is processed in such a way as to make it easy to digest. I know because I have had a hard time digesting many foods. I'm like the yellow canary they sent into the mines. If it died, the mine wasn't safe. I haven't died yet, but I've sure felt like it when I wasn't eating properly for my body!

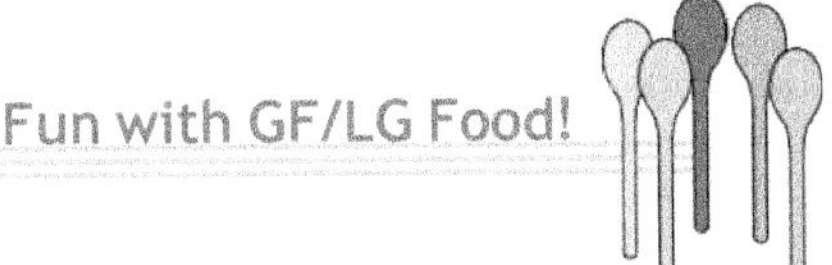

Celtic Sea Salt or Pink Himalayan Salt: The body needs salt! Some people are unbalanced in their sodium to potassium ratio. I know because I was one of them, even though I thought I ate a normal amount of salt. Think of how animals go for salt licks. Animals know how to eat what they need.
You need to check with your doctor if you feel there is a need to eat more or less salt, but please check with one who really knows.

Himalayan salt is preferable, since it is 450 million years old and has pure, ancient minerals that taste wonderful and are much easier for the body to assimilate. The Celtic sea salt has more minerals and is not processed like typical salt. One reason many people cannot eat salt is due to the chemicals used in processing common table salt.

Cow's Milk Products (some): Even though cow's milk is acid and not easy to digest for many of us, if the products are mostly fat, like cream or cream cheese, most people can eat them once in a while, but mainly if the products are organic and minimally processed. If you can get milk products raw from a local legally approved dairy it's better. But before you cheat, check with your doctor!

Goat Milk Products: Goat milk is more alkalizing than cow's milk, which helps the body heal. Try to get goat milk from a local, legally approved dairy, raw if possible.

Ghee: This is clarified Butter, available already made in health food stores (not so easy to make properly yourself—that's why I don't give recipe for it). Ghee has little or no effect on most people who are sensitive to dairy, while it has all the flavor of butter in spades. It's actually a more intense butter flavor. People who are allergic to cow's milk should use caution, as they may react to ghee.

Good Oils: The body needs oil, especially the nervous system and digestive system (for elimination). Oil has gotten a bad rap, but now it's getting it's due again, as folks are reading studies and learning how important good, healthy oils are, especially when not heated. High-heat oils, such as organic and cold-pressed, virgin grape seed oil, organic and cold-pressed virgin coconut oil, organic and cold-pressed, virgin high heat sunflower oil can be heated. Some people may not need as much oil as others. For example, my body type needs 40% oil and fat in my diet!

Important Note: Olive oil should *not* be used for cooking, as it has a very low flash point and turns rancid quickly.

Quinoa and Amaranth: These higher-protein, low glycemic grains were primary sources of sustenance for ancient people. They may give you added strength, and you will certainly not have the high-glycemic effects of rice or other grains. Millet is a good alternative, but has been cross-contaminated so that it may be no longer safe for Celiacs.

Sweet Leaf Stevia: This is a brand name stevia I recommend because it is minimally processed, even the liquid form.
When you can, I suggest using the powdered leaf itself, available in the bulk herb section of most health food stores. It doesn't matter what brand you use for the powdered leaf, as far as I know, as long as it's certified organic. Aside from the wonderful fact that stevia is a completely non-glycemic sweetener, I love the fact that it's supposed to actually be good for your pancreas! Yay!

Notes

Index

Note: Numbers in parentheses () are alternate pages.

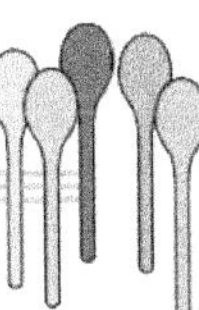

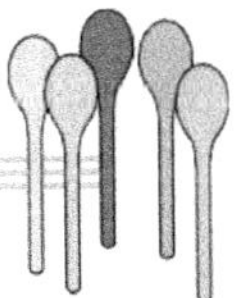

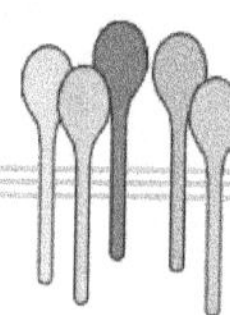

About the Author, Debbie Johnson

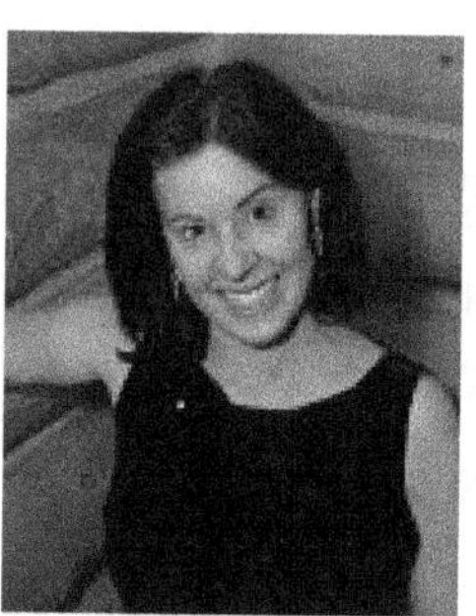

Debbie Johnson is the former owner and executive chef of
The Golden Chalice Restaurant and Gallery,
a 100% gluten-free, sugar-free, low-glycemic, organic, allergy-friendly establishment.
She's always loved cooking and creating delicious treats for special diets.

Debbie Johnson is also a best-selling author.
See *https://debbiejohnsonbooks.com* for a full list of her books.
The most popular is *Think Yourself Thin*.

DEBBIE'S OTHER BOOKS

- *Think Yourself Thin*
- *Think Yourself There*
- *Think Yourself Young*
- *Loving Relationships: Insights into Spirit*
- *Forget Willpower: Have Fun Family Fitness with Focused Imagination*

DEBBIE'S BOOKS OF A DIFFERENT GENRE

- *Dreams, Your Window to Heaven*
- *Exploring Past Lives to Heal the Present*
- *Soul Travel to Find God's Love*

www.ingramcontent.com/pod-product-compliance
Lightning Source LLC
Chambersburg PA
CBHW080914260726
48661CB00009B/3659